VIRTUAL SCREENING

Edited by **Mutasem O. Taha**

Virtual Screening
Edited by Mutasem O. Taha

Published by InTech
Janeza Trdine 9, 51000 Rijeka, Croatia

Publishing Process Manager Jana Sertic

Technical Editor Teodora Smiljanic

Cover Designer InTech Design Team

Additional hard copies can be obtained from orders@intechopen.com

Virtual Screening, Edited by Mutasem O. Taha
p. cm.
ISBN 978-953-51-0308-0

For EU product safety concerns:
IN TECH d.o.o., Prolaz Marije Krucifikse Kozulić 3, 51000 Rijeka, Croatia,
info@intechopen.com or visit our website at intechopen.com.

Meet the editor

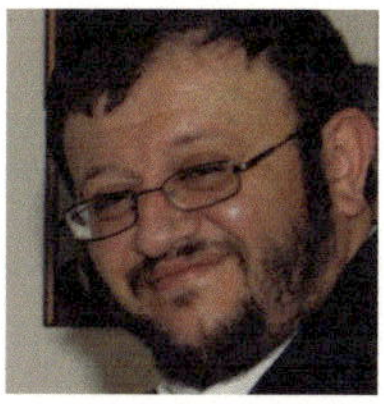

Dr Mutasem O. Taha is a Professor of medicinal chemistry and drug design at the Department of Pharmaceutical Sciences at the Faculty of Pharmacy/University of Jordan. He received his Pharmacy B.Sc. degree from The University of Jordan in 1992. In 1994 and 1998, he earned his M.Sc. and Ph.D. degrees, respectively, in Medicinal Chemistry from Loughborough University of Technology /United Kingdom. In 1998, he was appointed as assistant professor at the faculty of pharmacy/The University of Jordan. He was promoted to associate professor in 2003 and to full professor in 2008. Currently, he is interested in the areas of developing new polymeric materials for drug delivery and applications of molecular modeling techniques in drug design and pharmaceutics. Prof. Taha is particularly interested in the development of novel ligand-based strategies for assessing molecular flexibility of binding sites of various interesting enzymes and receptors. He has special interest in cancer, diabetes and obesity. Currently, he is in charge of the Drug Discovery Unit at the Faculty of Pharmacy - University of Jordan. Dr. Taha published more than 65 articles in international, peer-reviewed high caliber journals and has 4 registered patents. He received several local and regional awards in appreciation of his scientific merits.

Contents

Preface

Recent advances in drug discovery allowed access to powerful technologies that have a prominent virtual screening component. One of the chief difficulties in using these technologies is their requirement for interdisciplinary expertise in physical sciences, life sciences, statistical analyses and computer science. Therefore, the purpose of Virtual Screening is to help facilitate the employment of these new technologies in the process of drug discovery.

This volume describes a group of virtual screening methods and techniques that are used currently in modern drug discovery. The first section describes mixing pharmacophore modeling with classical quantitative structure-activity relationship (QSAR) analysis as powerful combination to enrich bioactivity among virtual screening hits. The next part of the book tries to evaluate recent advances and future trends on the emerging promising role of graphics processing units (GPUs) as platforms for virtual screening-based drug discovery, in particular in molecular dynamics simulations. The latter parts of the book discuss several examples on the use of virtual screening methods based on combinations of pharmacophore modeling and Comparative Molecular Field Analysis (CoMFA) or Comparative Molecular Similarity Indices Analysis (CoMSIA) for the discovery of anticancer, anti-leshmanial and acetylcholineesterase inhibitory agents. In each chapter, every effort has been made to incorporate detailed procedures, including software and its use, related to these technologies.

Virtual Screening is directed to those interested in the different aspects of drug design that include academicians (pharmacists, chemists), and scientists at pharmaceutical companies.

In all, this book is designed to provide readers not only with the planned insightful overview of key topics, but also with the customary ample supply of unfailing reproducible step-by-step procedures for techniques described.

Dr. Mutasem O. Taha
Professor of Drug Design and Medicinal Chemistry, Dept. of Pharmaceutical Sciences,
Faculty of Pharmacy, University of Jordan,
Jordan

Part 1

Pharmacophore Modelling and QSAR – A Powerful Combination for Virtual Screening

1

Mixing Pharmacophore Modeling and Classical QSAR Analysis as Powerful Tool for Lead Discovery

Mutasem O. Taha
Dept. of Pharmaceutical Sciences, Faculty of Pharmacy, University of Jordan
Jordan

1. Introduction

Discovery of new bioactive leads for subsequent optimization into drugs is both time consuming and expensive process. Two main approaches are currently available for lead discovery, namely, high throughput (*in vitro*) screening and computer-aided virtual (*in silico*) screening. Normally, *in silico* techniques are implemented as pre-filters to enrich the success rates of high throughput screening campaigns.

Computer-aided lead discovery techniques can be divided into two main methodologies: (1) Structure-based and (2) ligand-based methods. Structure-based methods depend on the availability of three-dimensional (3D) structure for the targeted biomolecule (enzyme of receptor). The target structure is normally employed as template to design sterically and electronically complementary ligands. On the other hand, ligand-based methods rely on assessing physicochemical and structural similarities among potent ligands and try to discern ligands' structural features responsible for high affinities from those responsible for poor affinities. In other words, ligand-based methods rely completely on ligand factors to assess ligand-receptor affinities.

Structure-based drug design can be divided into two major methodologies: de novo and docking-based design. De novo design involves the use of algorithms that construct virtual ligands inside binding pockets.[1-3] On the other hand, docking involves fitting virtual ligands, usually from large virtual libraries, into targeted binding sites employing computer algorithms that rely on force fields to calculate attractive and repulsive interactions within virtual ligand-protein complexes.[1-4]

The 3D structures of targeted receptors or enzymes are generally obtained via X-ray crystallographic scattering, nuclear magnetic resonance (NMR) or homology modeling.[1-4] However, reliance on crystallographic structures represents a major problem for structure-based design. Crystallographic structures are limited by inadequate resolution[5] and crystallization-related artifacts of the ligand-protein complex.[6-8] Moreover, crystallographic structures generally ignore structural heterogeneity related to protein anisotropic motion and discrete conformational substrates.[9]

Moreover, molecular docking, which is basically a conformational sampling procedure in which various docked conformations are explored to identify the right one, can be very challenging problem given the degree of conformational flexibility at the ligand-macromolecular level.[10-12] Although docking programs employ diverse methodologies to evaluate different ligand conformations within binding pockets,[13-23] conformational sampling must be guided by scoring function(s) to evaluate the fitness between the protein and the ligand.[4,24-29] The final docked conformations are selected according to their scores. Unfortunately, the sheer complexity of the underlying ligand-receptor molecular interactions extremely complicate free energy calculations and undermine the ability of scoring functions to evaluate binding free energies correctly in order to rank different potential ligand–receptor complexes.[1,3,5-8,10,30,31,39]

In addition to deciding the optimal docking/scoring combination for a particular docking problem, the molecular modeler must decide whether to leave crystallographically explicit water molecules in the binding site or not prior to ligand docking.[32-37] Furthermore, the fact that crystallographic structures lack information on hydrogen atoms means that it should be appropriately assumed whether ionizable moieties embedded within the binding site exist in their ionized form or not.[36,38]

Additional to the previous problems, use of single protein conformation for designing new ligands ignores important dynamic aspects of protein-ligand binding. In particular, the "induced fit" effects are ignored.[40,41] Unfortunately, all current computational models directed towards assessing the flexibility of macromolecular binding sites (e.g., soft receptors[42,43]; few critical rotable degrees of freedom in the receptor binding site[43-48]; systematic conformer searches of amino acids' side chains at the binding site[49]; molecular dynamics and free energy calculations conducted on flexible enzyme[50,51]; use of multiple crystallographic receptor structures[43,52]) suffer from two major drawbacks. Firstly, their computational cost, which reduces their effectiveness in virtual screening and fast docking, and secondly, their complete reliance on crystallographic structures.

The drawbacks of structure-based methods prompted us to introduce an interesting and novel ligand-based approach as a tool for characterizing binding sites' flexibilities. This approach ignores the protein template and focuses completely on the ligand side. It is carried out over two subsequent stages. Firstly, the pharmacophoric space of the targeted enzyme is extensively explored utilizing the three-dimensional Quantitative Structure Activity Relationship (3D-QSAR) software program CATALYST. The resulting binding models (hundreds) are then in allowed to compete within the context of classical quantitative structure-activity relationship analyses (QSAR) employing genetic algorithm (GA) and multiple linear regression (MLR) analyses. This process selects optimal combination of orthogonal pharmacophores that best explain the observed bioactivities, i.e., best possible QSAR model. Such combination of binding pharmacophores should correspond to accessible binding modes available for ligands within a particular binding pocket.

We previously reported the successful use of this combination to probe the induced fit flexibilities of activated factor X[53] and towards the discovery of new inhibitory leads against glycogen synthase kinase-3β,[54] bacterial MurF,[55] protein tyrosine phosphatase,[56] DPP IV,[57] hormone sensitive lipase,[58] β-secretase,[59] influenza neuraminidase,[60] cholesteryl ester transfer protein,[61] cycline dependent kinase,[62] Heat shock protein,[63] estrogen receptor β,[64] β-D-Glucosidase,[65] and β-D-Galactosidase.[66]

The author intends in this chapter to discuss the basic theoretical principles of this successful ligand-based approach and to provide interested audiences with experimental details related to this approach.

The modeling process of this approach can be divided in the following steps:

2. Data mining and conformational coverage

Firstly, the literature is extensively surveyed to identify as many reported structurally diverse ligands against the selected target as possible. The collected compounds must satisfy two important prerequisites: (i) they should be all bioassayed by a single procedure. Consistency in bioassay is a major requirement for QSAR modeling as it is not possible to model bioactivity data generated via more than one bioassay procedure. (ii) They must exhibit wide bioactivity range, i.e., over > 4 logarthmic cycles.

Initially, the 2D structures of the inhibitors are imported into the modeling package (CATALYST) and converted automatically into plausible 3D single conformer representations and energy minimized to the closest local minimum. The resulting single conformer 3D structures are normally used as starting points for conformational analysis for pharmacophore modeling and in the determination of various molecular descriptors for QSAR modeling.

The conformational space of each ligand is extensively sampled usually utilizing the poling algorithm employed within the CONFIRM module of CATALYST.[67] Efficient conformational coverage guarantees minimum conformation-related noise during pharmacophore generation and validation stages because pharmacophore generation and pharmacophore-based search procedures are known for their sensitivity to inadequate conformational sampling within the training compounds.[60]

The logarithm of measured IC_{50}, EC_{50} or Ki values are used in pharmacophore modeling and QSAR analysis, thus correlating the data linear to the free energy change.

2.1 Exploration of pharmacophoric space

2.1.1 The algorithm

Normally we implement the HYPOGEN module within CATALYST package to explore the pharmacophoric space of different ligands. CATALYST-HYPOGEN enables automatic pharmacophore construction by using a collection of at least 16 molecules with bioactivities spanning over 3.5 orders of magnitude.[67]

CATALYST-HYPOGEN models drug-receptor interaction using information derived from the ligand structure. It identifies a 3D array of a maximum of five chemical features common to active training molecules, which provides a relative alignment for each input molecule consistent with their binding to a proposed common receptor site. The chemical features considered can be hydrogen bond donors and acceptors (HBDs and HBAs), aliphatic and aromatic hydrophobes (Hbic), positive and negative ionizable (PosIon and NegIon) groups and aromatic planes (RingArom). CATALYST pharmacophores have been used as 3D queries for database searching and in 3D-QSAR studies.[54-66]

Although pharmacophore modeling employing HYPOGEN has been heavily reviewed in the literature,[68-76] a brief discussion of this algorithm is provided herein to allow better readability of the chapter.

HYPOGEN pharmacophore exploration proceeds through three successive phases: the constructive phase, subtractive phase and optimization phase.[67-76]

During the constructive phase, CATALYST generates common conformational alignments among the most-active training compounds. Only molecular alignments based on a maximum of five chemical features are considered. The program identifies a particular compound as being within the most active category if it satisfies equation (1).[73]

$$(\text{MAct} \times \text{UncMAct}) - (\text{Act} / \text{UncAct}) > 0.0 \quad (1)$$

Where "MAct" is the activity of the most active compound in the training set, "Unc" is the uncertainty of the compounds and "Act" is the activity of the training compounds under question. However, if there are more than eight most-active inhibitors, only the top eight are used.

In the subsequent subtractive phase, CATALYST eliminates some hypotheses that fit inactive training compounds. A particular training compound is defined as being inactive if it satisfies equation (2): [67-76]

$$\text{Log}(\text{Act}) - \log(\text{MAct}) > 3.5 \quad (2)$$

However, in the optimization phase, CATALYST applies fine perturbations in the form of vectored feature rotation, adding new feature and/or removing a feature, to selected hypotheses that survived the subtractive phase, in an attempt to find new models of enhanced bioactivity/mapping correlation, i.e., improved 3D-QSAR properties.[67-76]

Eventually, CATALYST selects the highest-ranking models (10 by default) and presents them as the optimal pharmacophore hypotheses resulting from the particular automatic modeling run.

2.1.2 Selection of training subsets

The fact that pharmacophore modeling requires limited number of carefully selected training compounds (from 16-45 compounds only)[67-76] that exhibit bioactivity variations attributable solely to the presence or absence of pharmacophoric features, i.e., not due to steric or electronic factors, makes it impossible to explore the pharmacophore space of large training sets in one shot (e.g., we normally collect more that 100 compounds), partly because CATALYST-HYPOGEN is not suited to handle large number of compounds and partly because pharmacophore modeling is generally confused by electronic and steric bioactivity modifying factors commonly encountered in SAR data. This dilemma prompted us to break compound lists into smaller training subsets compatible with pharmacophore modeling, i.e., of bioactivity variations attributable solely to the presence or absence of pharmacophoric features. Nevertheless, the basic problem in this approach is to identify a particular training set capable of representing the whole list of collected compounds. This problem can be very significant in cases of large SAR lists. We found that the best way to solve this problem is by exploring the pharmacophoric space of several carefully selected training subsets, i.e., from the whole list of collected compounds, followed by allowing the resulting pharmacophores to compete within the context of genetic function approximation-based quantitative structure-activity relationship (GFA-QSAR) analysis such that the best pharmacophore(s) capable of explaining bioactivity variations across the whole list of collected compounds is(are) selected. However, since pharmacophore models fail in explaining electronic and steric bioactivity-modulating effects, the GFA-QSAR process should be allowed to select other 2D physicochemical descriptors to complement the selected pharmacophore(s) (see below).

The training compounds in these subsets are selected in such away to guarantee maximal 3D diversity and continuous bioactivity spread over more than 3.5 logarithmic cycles. Moreover, training subsets are selected in such a way that their member compounds share certain apparent 3D SAR rules (by visual evaluation).

We usually give special emphasis to the 3D diversity of the most active compounds in each training subset because of their significant influence on the extent of the evaluated pharmacophoric space during the constructive phase of HYPOGEN algorithm. However, it must be mentioned that not all collected compounds are incorporated in the pharmacophore training subsets, in fact, compounds that exhibit limited diversity or significant bioactivity-modifying steric or electronic influences are excluded from the training subsets.

2.1.3 Modeling boundaries

HYPOGEN implements an optimization algorithm that evaluates large number of potential binding models for a particular target through fine perturbations to hypotheses that survived the constructive and subtractive phases of the modeling algorithm.[67-76] The extent of the evaluated pharmacophoric space is reflected by the configuration (Config.) cost calculated for each modeling run. It is generally recommended that the Config. cost of any HYPOGEN run not to exceed 17 (corresponding to 2^{17} hypotheses to be assessed by HYPOGEN) to guarantee thorough analysis of all models.[71-73] The size of the investigated pharmacophoric space is a function of training compounds, selected input chemical features and other CATALYST control parameters.[67-76]

We envisaged that restricting the size of explored pharmacophoric space should improve the efficiency of optimization via allowing efficient assessment of limited number of pharmacophoric models. On the other hand, extreme restrictions imposed on the evaluated pharmacophoric space might reduce the possibility of discovering optimal binding hypotheses, as they might occur outside the "boundaries" of the evaluated space.

Therefore, we normally explore the pharmacophoric space of targeted ligands under reasonably imposed "boundaries" through numerous HYPOGEN runs and employing several carefully selected training subsets.

Guided by our rationally restricted pharmacophoric exploration concept, we usually restrict HYPOGEN to explore pharmacophoric models incorporating limited number of features, e.g., from zero to one negative NegIon, or PosIon features or from zero to three HBA, Hbic, and RingArom features instead of the default range of zero to five. Furthermore, we normally instructed HYPOGEN to explore only 4- and 5-featured pharmacophores, i.e., ignore models of lesser number of features in order to further narrow the investigated pharmacophoric space and to better represent the diverse interactions between known ligands and binding pockets. In fact, three- and two-featured pharmacophores are rather promiscuous as 3D search queries and not adequate descriptions of ligand-receptor binding.

2.1.4 Assessment of generated pharmacophore models

When generating hypotheses, CATALYST attempts to minimize a cost function consisting of three terms: Weight cost, Error cost and Configuration cost.[67-76] Weight cost is a value that increases as the feature weight in a model deviates from an ideal value of 2. The deviation between the estimated activities of the training set and their experimentally determined values adds to the error cost. The activity of any compound can be estimated from a particular hypothesis through equation (3).[73]

$$\text{Log (Estimated Activity)} = \text{I} + \text{Fit} \qquad (3)$$

Where, I = the intercept of the regression line obtained by plotting the log of the biological activity of the training set compounds against the Fit values of the training compounds. The Fit value for any compound is obtained automatically employing equation (4).[73]

$$\text{Fit} = \Sigma \text{ mapped hypothesis features} \times W\,[1-\Sigma\,(\text{disp/tol})^2] \qquad (4)$$

Where, Σ mapped hypothesis features represents the number of pharmacophore features that successfully superimpose (i.e., map or overlap with) corresponding chemical moieties within the fitted compound, W is the weight of the corresponding hypothesis feature spheres. This value is fixed to 1.0 in CATALYST-generated models. disp is the distance between the center of a particular pharmacophoric sphere (feature centroid) and the center of the corresponding superimposed chemical moiety of the fitted compound; tol is the radius of the pharmacophoric feature sphere (known as Tolerance, equals to 1.6 Å by default). $\Sigma\,(\text{disp/tol})^2$ is the summation of $(\text{disp/tol})^2$ values for all pharmacophoric features that successfully superimpose corresponding chemical functionalities in the fitted compound.[67-76]

The third cost term, i.e., the configuration cost, penalizes the complexity of the hypothesis. This is a fixed cost, which is equal to the entropy of the hypothesis space. The more the numbers of features (a maximum of five) in a generated hypothesis, the higher is the entropy with subsequent increase in this cost. The overall cost (total cost) of a hypothesis is calculated by summing over the three cost factors. However, error cost is the main contributor to the total cost.

CATALYST also calculates the cost of the null hypothesis, which presumes that there is no relationship in the data and that experimental activities are normally distributed about their mean. Accordingly, the greater the difference from the null hypothesis cost, the more likely that the hypothesis does not reflect a chance correlation. In a successful automatic modeling run, CATALYST ranks the generated models according to their total costs.[67-76]

An additional approach to assess the quality of CATALYST-HYPOGEN pharmacophores is to cross-validate them using the Cat-Scramble module implemented in CATALYST. This validation procedure is based on Fisher's randomization test.[43] In this validation test, a 95% confidence level was selected, which instruct CATALYST to generate 19 random spreadsheets by the Cat-Scramble command. Subsequently, CATALYST-HYPOGEN is challenged to use these random spreadsheets to generate hypotheses using exactly the same features and parameters used in generating the initial unscrambled hypotheses.[67] Success in generating pharmacophores of comparable cost criteria to those produced by the original unscrambled data reduces the confidence in the training compounds and the unscrambled original pharmacophore models.

Eventually, the top 10 binding hypotheses (i.e., pharmacophores) from each automatic HYPOGEN run are automatically ranked according to their corresponding "total cost" values and presented as output of the HYPOGEN run.

2.2 Clustering of successful pharmacophore hypotheses

Because the number of generated pharmacophores during our pharmacophore exploration step is usually large (> 60 model) and they usually share several 3D features and properties (cost criteria, Cat.scramble confidence, etc …), we normally cluster the resulting models into limited number of groups (10-30) utilizing the hierarchical average linkage method available in CATALYST. The highest-ranking hypothesis within each cluster (i.e., of lowest cost or highest correlation with bioactivity of the whole collected list) is selected to represent the corresponding cluster in subsequent QSAR modeling.

Clustering aims at avoiding overloading genetic function approximation-multiple linear regression (GFA-MLR), implemented during QSAR modeling, with numerous independent variables, which may allow the emergence of less-than-optimal regression models.

2.3 QSAR modeling

Pharmacophoric hypotheses are important tools in drug design and discovery as they provide excellent insights into ligand-macromolecule recognition and they can be used to mine for new biologically interesting scaffolds. However, their predictive value as 3D-QSAR models is usually limited by steric shielding and bioactivity-enhancing or -reducing auxiliary groups.[76] This point combined with the fact that pharmacophore exploration usually furnish several binding hypotheses of comparable success criteria and 3D features prompt us to use classical QSAR analysis to search for optimal combination of pharmacophore(s) and other 2D descriptors capable of explaining bioactivity variation across the whole list of collected inhibitors. We normally employ genetic function approximation and multiple linear regression QSAR (GFA-MLR-QSAR) analysis to search for an optimal QSAR equation(s) using the logarithm of measured $1/IC_{50}$ or $1/Ki$ values are as dependent variables (thus correlating the data linear to the free energy change).

GFA-MLR-QSAR selects optimal descriptor combinations based on the Darwinian concept of genetic evolution whereby the statistical criteria of regression models from different descriptor combinations (chromosomes) are employed as fitness criteria.[77] GFA-MLR-QSAR analysis is employed to explore various combinations of pharmacophores and other structural descriptors and to evaluate their statistical properties as predictive QSAR models.

Representative pharmacophore hypotheses (selected during the clustering stage) are fitted against all collected ligands and their fit values (determined by equation 4) are enrolled, together with other 2D and 1D structural descriptors, as independent variables (genes) in a cycle of GFA-MLR-QSAR analysis over thousands of iterations.[77]

Other structural descriptors include various simple and valence connectivity indices, electro-topological state indices and other molecular descriptors (e.g., logarithm of partition coefficient, polarizability, dipole moment, molecular volume, molecular weight, molecular surface area, etc.).[77]

However, to assess the predictive power of the optimal QSAR models on external set of inhibitors, we usually randomly select around 20% of the collected ligands and employ them as external testing molecules for validating optimal QSAR model(s) (r^2_{PRESS}). Moreover, all QSAR models are cross-validated automatically using the leave-one-out cross-validation.[77]

Emergence of two or more orthogonal pharmacophoric models in the optimal QSAR model suggests the existence of complementary two or more corresponding binding modes accessible to ligands within the binding pocket of target protein, i.e., one of the pharmacophores can optimally explain the bioactivities of some training inhibitors, while the others explain the remaining inhibitors. Such conclusions were reached about the binding pockets of several targets, e.g., factor Xa, GSK-3β, and Mur F.[57-63]

2.4 Final validation of optimal QSAR model and associated pharmacophores

To establish the validity of optimal GFA-selected QSAR model and associated pharmacophore(s), we normally implement two validation methods: (1) Receiver-Operating Characteristic (ROC) curve analysis, and (2) Comparing QSAR-selected pharmacophore(s) with the corresponding binding site, however, this is only done upon having available crystallographic structure of the targeted receptor.

2.4.1 Receiver Operating Characteristic (ROC) curve analysis

In ROC analysis, the ability of a particular pharmacophore model to correctly classify a list of compounds as actives or inactives is indicated by the area under the curve (AUC) of the corresponding ROC as well as other parameters, namely, overall accuracy, overall specificity, overall true positive rate and overall false negative rate.[78-79]

The testing list for ROC analyses are usually prepared as described by Verdonk and co-workers.[78] Briefly, decoy compounds are selected based on three basic one-dimensional (1D) properties that allow the assessment of distance (D) between two molecules (e.g., i and j): (1) the number of hydrogen-bond donors (NumHBD); (2) number of hydrogen-bond acceptors (NumHBA) and (3) count of nonpolar atoms (NP, defined as the summation of Cl, F, Br, I, S and C atoms in a particular molecule). For each active compound in the test set, the distance to the nearest other active compound is assessed by their Euclidean Distance (Equation 5):

$$D(i,j)=\sqrt{(NumHBD_i - NumHBD_j)^2 + (NumHBA_i - NumHBA_j)^2 + (NP_i - NP_j)^2} \qquad (5)$$

The minimum distances are then averaged over all active compounds (Dmin). Subsequently, for each active compound in the test set, around 40 decoys are randomly chosen from the ZINC database.[80] The decoys are selected in such a way that they did not exceed Dmin distance from their corresponding active compound.

To diversify active members in the list, we exclude any active compound having zero distance ($D(i,j)$) from other active compound(s) in the test set.

The test set is then screened by each particular pharmacophore employing the "Best flexible search" option implemented in CATALYST, while the conformational spaces of the compounds are usually generated employing the "Fast conformation generation option" implemented in CATALYST. Compounds missing one or more features were discarded from the hit list. *In-silico* hits were scored employing their fit values as calculated by equation (4).

The ROC curve analysis describes the sensitivity (Se or true positive rate, equation 6) for any possible change in the number of selected compounds (n) as a function of (1-Sp). Sp is defined as specificity or true negative rate (equation 7).[79,81]

$$Se = \frac{Number\ of\ Selected\ Actives}{Total\ Number\ of\ Actives} = \frac{TP}{TP + FN} \tag{6}$$

$$Sp = \frac{Number\ of\ Discarded\ Inactives}{Total\ Number\ of\ Inactives} = \frac{TN}{TN + FP} \tag{7}$$

where, TP is the number of active compounds captured by the virtual screening method (true positives), FN is the number of active compounds discarded by the virtual screening method, TN is the number of discarded decoys (presumably inactives), while FP is the number of captured decoys (presumably inactive).[79,81]

If all molecules scored by a virtual screening (VS) protocol with sufficient discriminatory power are ranked according to their score (i.e., fit values), starting with the best-scored molecule and ending with the molecule that got the lowest score, most of the actives will have a higher score than the decoys. Since some of the actives will be scored lower than decoys, an overlap between the distribution of active molecules and decoys will occur, which will lead to the prediction of false positives and false negatives.[79,81] The selection of one score value as a threshold strongly influences the ratio of actives to decoys and therefore the validation of a VS method. The ROC curve method avoids the selection of a threshold by considering all Se and Sp pairs for each score threshold.[79,81] A ROC curve is plotted by setting the score of the active molecule as the first threshold. Afterwards, the number of decoys within this cutoff is counted and the corresponding Se and Sp pair is calculated. This calculation is repeated for the active molecule with the second highest score and so forth, until the scores of all actives are considered as selection thresholds.

The ROC curve representing ideal distributions, where no overlap between the scores of active molecules and decoys exists, proceeds from the origin to the upper-left corner until all the actives are retrieved and Se reaches the value of 1. In contrast to that, the ROC curve for a set of actives and decoys with randomly distributed scores tends towards the Se = 1-Sp line asymptotically with increasing number of actives and decoys.[79,81] The success of a particular virtual screening workflow can be judged from the following criteria:

1. Area under the ROC curve (AUC).[79,81] In an optimal ROC curve an AUC value of 1 is obtained; however, random distributions cause an AUC value of 0.5. Virtual screening that performs better than a random discrimination of actives and decoys retrieve an

AUC value between 0.5 and 1, whereas an AUC value lower than 0.5 represents the unfavorable case of a virtual screening method that has a higher probability to assign the best scores to decoys than to actives.[79,81]

2. Overall Accuracy (ACC): describes the percentage of correctly classified molecules by the screening protocol (equation 8). Testing compounds are assigned a binary score value of zero (compound not captured) or one (compound captured).[79,81]

$$ACC = \frac{TP + TN}{N} = \frac{A}{N}.Se + \left(1 - \frac{A}{N}\right).Sp \qquad (8)$$

where, N is the total number of compounds in the testing database, A is the number of true actives in the testing database.

3. Overall specificity (SPC): describes the percentage of discarded inactives by the particular virtual screening workflow. Inactive test compounds are assigned a binary score value of zero (compound not captured) or one (compound captured) regardless to their individual fit values.[79,81]
4. Overall True Positive Rate (TPR or overall sensitivity): describes the fraction percentage of captured actives from the total number of actives. Active test compounds are assigned a binary score value of zero (compound not captured) or one (compound captured) regardless to their individual fit values.[79,81]
5. Overall False Negative Rate (FNR or overall percentage of discarded actives): describes the fraction percentage of active compounds discarded by the virtual screening method. Discarded active test compounds are assigned a binary score value of zero (compound not captured) or one (compound captured) regardless to their individual fit values.[79,81]

2.5 *In Silico* screening

Eventually, optimal QSAR-selected pharmacophores are employed as 3D search queries against several electronic multiconformer structural databases (e.g. NCI 238,819 structures) using the "Best Flexible Database Search" option implemented within CATALYST. Compounds that have their chemical groups spatially overlap (map) with corresponding features of the particular pharmacophoric model are captured as hits. Hits are normally filtered based on Lipinski's and Veber's rules.[82,83] Surviving hits are then fitted against QSAR-selected pharmacophores and their fit values, together with other relevant molecular descriptors, are substituted in optimal QSAR equation to predict their bioactivities. The highest-ranking available hits are evaluated *in vitro*.

Usually, the acquired hits are screened at 10 μM concentrations, subsequently; compounds of significant bioactivities at 10 μM are further assessed to determine their IC_{50} values.

It remains to be mentioned that although QSAR predictions are rather accurate with some hit compounds, experimental IC_{50} values of other hits differ significantly from QSAR predictions. These errors appear are usually related to structural differences between training compounds used in QSAR and pharmacophore modeling compared to hit molecules. This discrepancy seems to limit the extrapolatory potential of the QSAR equation.

3. Conclusions

This chapter summarizes an interesting novel approach for the discovery of new bioactive leads by implementing a sequential process of pharmacophore modeling and QSAR analysis. This approach has been used for the discovery of potent inhibitors against at least a dozen enzymes and receptors.

4. References

[1] Song, C. M.; Lim, S. J.; Tong, J. C. R. *Brief Bioinform.* 2009, 10, 579-591.
[2] Menikarachchi, L. C.; Gascon, J. A. *Curr. Top. Med. Chem.* 2010, 10, 46–54.
[3] Jorgensen, W. L. *Acc. Chem. Res.* 2009, 42, 724–733.
[4] Hecht, D.; Fogel, G. B. *Curr. Comput.-Aided Drug Des.* 2009, 5, 56–68.
[5] Beeley, N. R. A.; Sage, C. *Targets* 2003, 2, 19–25.
[6] Klebe, G. *Drug Discovery Today* 2006, 11, 580–594.
[7] Steuber, H.; Zentgraf, M.; Gerlach, C.; Sotriffer, C. A.; Heine, A; Klebe, G. *J. Mol. Biol.* 2006, 363, 174–187.
[8] Stubbs, M. T.; Reyda, S.; Dullweber, F.; Moller, M.; Klebe, G.; Dorsch, D.; Mederski, W.; Wurziger, H. *ChemBioChem* 2002, 3, 246–249.
[9] DePristo, M. A.; de Bakker, P. I. W.; Blundell, T. L. *Structure* 2004, 12, 831–838.
[10] Morris, G. M.; Olson, A. J.; Goodsell, D. S. *Princ. Med. Chem.* 2000, 8, 31–48.
[11] Kontoyianni, M.; McClellan, L. M.; Sokol, G. S. *J. Med. Chem.* 2004, 47, 558–565.
[12] Beier, C.; Zacharias, M. *Expert Opin. Drug Dis.* 2010, 5, 347–359.
[13] Rarey, M.; Kramer, B.; Lengauer, T.; Klebe, G. *J. Mol. Biol.* 1996, 261, 470–489.
[14] Ewing, T. J. A.; Makino, S.; Skillman, A. G.; Kuntz, I. D. *J. Comput. Aid Mol. Des.* 2001, 15, 411–428.
[15] Jones, G.; Willett, P.; Glen, R. C.; Leach, A. R.; Taylor, R. *J. Mol. Biol.* 1997, 267, 727–748.
[16] Vaque, M.; Ardrevol, A.; Blade, C.; Salvado, M. J; Blay, M.; Fernandez-Larrea, J.; Arola, L.; Pujadas, G. *Curr. Pharm. Anal.* 2008, 4, 1–19.
[17] Cosconati, S.; Forli, S.; Perryman, A. L.; Harris, R.; Goodsell, D. S.; Olson, A. J. *Expert Opin. Drug Dis.* 2010, 5, 597–607.
[18] Morris, G. M.; Goodsell, D. S.; Halliday, R. S.; Huey, R.; Hart, W. E.; Belew, R. K.; Olson, A. J. *J. Comput. Chem.* 1998, 19, 1639-1662.
[19] Halgren, T. A.; Murphy, R. B.; Friesner, R. A.; Beard, H. S.; Frye, L. L.; Pollard, W. T.; Banks, J. L. *J. Med. Chem.* 2004, 47, 1750–1759.
[20] CERIUS2 LigandFit, version 4.10; Accelrys, Inc.: San Diego, 2000.
[21] FRED, version 2.1; OpenEye Scientific Software: Santa Fe, NM, 2006.
[22] Diller, D. J.; Merz, K. M. *Proteins* 2001, 43, 113–124.
[23] Rao, S. N.; Head, M. S.; Kulkarni, A.; LaLonde, J. M. *J. Chem. Inf. Model.* 2007, 47, 2159-2171.
[24] Bissantz, C.; Folkers, G.; Rognan, D. *J. Med. Chem.* 2000, 43, 4759–4767.
[25] Gao, W. R.; Lai, Y. L. *J. Mol. Model.* 1998, 4, 379–394.
[26] Krammer, A.; Kirchhoff, P. D.; Jiang, X.; Venkatachalam, C. M.; Waldman, M. *J. Mol. Graphics Modell.* 2005, 23, 395–407.
[27] Velec, H. F. G.; Gohlke, H.; Klebe, G. *J. Med. Chem.* 2005, 48, 6296–6303.

[28] Jain, A. N. *Curr. Protein Pept. Sci.* 2006, 7, 407–20.
[29] Rajamani, R.; Good, A. C. *Curr. Opin. Drug Discovery Dev.* 2007, 10, 308–15.
[30] Tame, J. R. H. *J. Comput.-Aided Mol. Des.* 1999, 13, 99–108.
[31] Kollman, P. *Chem. Rev.* 1993, 93, 2395–2417.
[32] Homans, S. W. *Drug Discovery Today* 2007, 12, 534–539.
[33] Poornima, C. S.; Dean, P. M. *J. Comput.-Aided Mol. Des.* 1995, 9, 500–512.
[34] Poornima, C. S.; Dean, P. M. *J. Comput.-Aided Mol. Des.* 1995, 9, 513–520.
[35] Poornima, C. S.; Dean, P. M. *J. Comput.-Aided Mol. Des.* 1995, 9, 521–531.
[36] Koehler, K. F.; Rao, S. N.; Snyder, J. P. Modeling drug-receptor interactions. In Guidebook on Molecular Modeling in Drug Design; Cohen, N. C., Ed.; Academic Press; San Diego, 1996; pp 235-336.
[37] Pastor, M.; Cruciani, G.; Watson, K. *J. Med. Chem.* 1997, 40, 4089–4102.
[38] Silverman, R. A. The Organic Chemistry of Drug Design and Drug Action; Academic Press: San Diego, 1991, pp 62-65.
[39] Krissinel, E. *J. Comput. Chem.* 2009, 31, 133–143.
[40] D. E. Koshland, *Proc. Natl Acad. Sci. USA* 1958, 44, 98-104.
[41] W.L. Jorgensen, Science 254 (1991) 951-955.
[42] Cohen N. C., Guidebook on Molecular Modeling in Drug Design, Academic Press, UK, 1996.
[43] M. L. Teodoro, L. E. Kavraki, *Curr. Pharm. Design* 2003, 9, 1635-1648.
[44] R. L. Dunbrack, M. Karplus, *J. Mol. Biol.* 1993, 230, 543-574.
[45] G. Vriend, C. Sander, P. F. W. Stouten, *Prot. Eng.* 1994, 7 23-29.
[46] H. Shrauber, F. Eisenhaber, P. Argos, *J. Mol. Biol.* 1993, 230 592-612.
[47] A. R. Leach, I. D. Kuntz, *J. Comput. Chem.* 1992, 13, 730-748.
[48] R. Leach, *J. Mol. Biol.* 1994, 235, 345-356.
[49] F. Eisenmenger, P. Argos, R. Abagyan, *J. Mol. Biol.* 1993, 231 849-860.
[50] P. Kollman, Curr. Opin. Struct. Biol. 4 (1994) 240-245.
[51] McCammon, J. A., Harvey, S. C., Dynamics of Proteins and Nucleic Acids, Cambridge University Press, Cambridge, 1987.
[52] R. M. A. Knegtel, I. D. Kuntz, C. M. Oshiro, *J. Mol. Biol.* 1997, 266 , 424-440.
[53] Taha, Mutasem O.; Qandil, Amjad M.; Zaki, Dhia D.; Murad A. AlDamen. *Eur. J. Med. Chem.* 2005, 40, 701-727.
[54] Taha, M.O.; Bustanji, Y.; Al-Ghussein, M.A.S.; Mohammad, M.; Zalloum, H.; Al-Masri, I.M.; Atallah, N. *J. Med. Chem.* 2008, 51, 2062-2077.
[55] Taha, M.O.; Atallah, N.; Al-Bakri, A.G.; Paradis-Bleau, C.; Zalloum, H.; Younis, K.; Levesque, R.C. *Bioorg. Med. Chem.* 2008, 16, 1218-1235.
[56] Taha, M.O.; Bustanji, Y.; Al-Bakri, A.G.; Yousef, M.; Zalloum, W.A.; Al-Masri, I.M.; Atallah, N. *J. Mol. Graphics Modell.* 2007, 25, 870–884.
[57] Al-masri, I.M.; Mohammad, M. K.; Taha, M.O. *ChemMedChem* 2008, 3, 1763–1779.
[58] Taha, M.O.; Dahabiyeh, L. A.; Bustanji, Y.; Zalloum, H.; Saleh, S. *J. Med. Chem.* 2008, 51, 6478–6494.
[59] Al-Nadaf, A.; Abu Sheikha, G.; Taha, M.O. *Bioorg. Med. Chem.* 2010, 18, 3088-115.
[60] Abu-Hammad, A. M.; Taha, M.O. *J. Chem. Inf. Model.* 2009, 49, 978–996.

[61] Abu Khalaf, R.; Abu Sheikha, G; Bustanji, Y.; Taha, M.O. *Eur. J. Med. Chem.* 2010, 45, 1598–1617.

[62] Al-Sha'er, M.; Taha, M.O. *Eur. J. Med. Chem.* 2010, 45, 4316–4330.

[63] Al-Sha'er, M.; Taha, M.O. *J. Chem. Inf. Model.* 2010, 50, 1706–1723.

[64] Taha, M.O.; Trarairah, M.; Zalloum, H.; Abu Sheikha G. *J. Mol. Graph Model.*, 2010, 28, 383-400.

[65] Abu Khalaf, R.; Abdula, A.; Mubarak, M.; Taha, M. *J. Mol. Model.* 2011, 17, 443–464.

[66] Abdula, A.; Abu Khalaf, R.; Mubarak, M.; Taha, M. *J. Comput. Chem.* 2011, 3, 463–482.

[67] CATALYST 4.11 Users' Manual (2005) Accelrys Software Inc San Diego, CA.

[68] Poptodorov K, Luu T, Langer T, Hoffmann R (2006) In: Hoffmann R D (ed) Methods and Principles in Medicinal Chemistry. Pharmacophores and Pharmacophores Searches Wiley-VCH, Weinheim, Germany

[69] Li H, Sutter J, Hoffmann R (2000) In: Güner O F (ed) Pharmacophore Perception Development and Use in Drug Design, International University Line, La Jolla, CA.

[70] Sutter J, Güner O, Hoffmann R, Li H, Waldman M (2000) In: Güner O F (ed) Pharmacophore Perception Development and Use in Drug Design, International University Line, La Jolla, CA.

[71] Discovery Studio version 25 (DS 25) User Manual (2009) Accelrys Inc, San Diego, CA

[72] Sutter J, Güner O, Hoffmann R, Li H, Waldman M (2000) In: Güner O F (ed) Pharmacophore Perception Development and Use in Drug Design, International University Line, La Jolla, CA.

[73] Kurogi Y, Güner O F (2001) Curr Med Chem 8: 1035–1055

[74] Poptodorov K, Luu T, Langer T, Hoffmann R (2006) In: Hoffmann R D (ed) Methods and Principles in Medicinal Chemistry Pharmacophores and Pharmacophores Searches, Wiley-VCH, Weinheim, Germany.

[75] Li H, Sutter J, Hoffmann R (2000) In: Güner O F (ed) Pharmacophore Perception Development and Use in Drug Design, International University Line: La Jolla, CA.

[76] Bersuker I B, Bahçeci S, Boggs JE (2000) In: Güner O F (ed) Pharmacophore Perception Development and Use in Drug Design, International University Line: La Jolla, CA.

[77] CERIUS2, QSAR Users' Manual, version 4.10; Accelrys Inc.: San Diego, CA, 2005; pp 43-88, 221-235.

[78] M.L. Verdonk, V. Berdini, M.J. Hartshorn, W.T.M. Mooij, C.W. Murray, R.D. Taylor, P. Watson *J. Chem. Inf. Model.*. 2004, 44, 793-806.

[79] J. Kirchmair, P. Markt, S. Distinto, G. Wolber, T. Langer, *J. Comput.-Aided Mol. Des.* 2008, 22, 213-228.

[80] J.J. Irwin, B.K. Shoichet, *J. Chem. Inf. Model.* 2004, 45, 177-182.

[81] N. Triballeau, F. Acher, I. Brabet, J.-P. Pin, H.-O. Bertrand, *J. Med. Chem.* 2005, 48, 2534-2547.

[82] C.A. Lipinski, F. Lombardo, B.W. Dominy, P.J. Feeney. *Adv. Drug Del. Reviews*, 2001, 46, 3-26.

[83] D.F. Veber, S.R. Johnson, H.-Y. Cheng, B.R. Smith, K.W. Ward, K.D. Kopple, *J. Med. Chem.* 2002, 45, 2615-2623.

Part 2

GPUs in Virtual Screening – Current State and Future Perspectives

2

Recent Advances and Future Trend on the Emerging Role of GPUs as Platforms for Virtual Screening-Based Drug Discovery

Horacio Pérez-Sánchez, José M. Cecilia and José M. García
Computer Engineering Dept., University of Murcia
Spain

1. Introduction

Virtual Screening (VS) has played an important role in drug discovery, and experimental techniques are increasingly complemented by numerical simulation (Schneider & Böhm, 2002). Although VS methods have been investigated for many years and several compounds could be identified that evolved into drugs, the impact of VS has not yet fulfilled all expectations. Neither the docking methods nor the scoring functions used presently are sufficiently accurate to reliably identify high-affinity ligands. To deal with a large number of potential candidates (many databases comprise hundreds of thousands of ligands), VS methods must be very fast and yet identify "the needles in the haystack". In many VS applications the predicted ligands turn out to have low affinity (false positives), while high affinity ligands rank low in the database (false negatives). In contrast, established simulation (not scoring) methods, such as free-energy perturbation theory, can determine relative changes in the affinity when ligands are changed slightly (group substitutions). However, these techniques require hundreds of CPU hours for each ligand, while simulation strategies to compute absolute binding affinities require thousands of CPU hours for each ligand (Wang et al., 2006). In comparison to these techniques, VS methods must make significant approximations regarding the affinity calculation and the sampling of possible receptor complex conformations. These approximations would be justifiable, as long as the relative order of affinity is preserved at the high-affinity end of the database.

Nowadays there are several receptor based VS methods available, including AutoDock (Zhang et al., 2005), FlexX (Xing et al., 2004), Glide (Friesner & Banks, 2004), FlexScreen (Kokh & Wenzel, 2008), and ICM (Bursulaya et al., 2003), each of them having different technical features. Most modern methods use an atomistic representation of the protein and the ligand. They permit the exploration of thousands of possible binding poses and ligand conformations in the docking process. As a result, binding modes are predicted reliably for many complexes. In general, methods that permit continuous ligand flexibility are somewhat more accurate than those that select conformations from a finite ensemble. However, recent unbiased comparative evaluations of affinity estimations showed little correlation between measured and predicted affinities over a wide range of receptor-ligand complexes. As a result, enrichment rates remain poor for many methods. Since high-accuracy, but also high-cost simulation protocols for affinity calculations are available, one avenue to improve weaknesses of existing VS programs is to move into the direction of established all-atom biophysical simulation. Both better scoring functions and novel docking strategies will contribute in this direction.

But one of the main problems in this direction is that all VS methods mentioned previously were developed for and run on commodity PCs, with its limitations in terms of availability of computing power. However, current PCs are becoming powerful desktop machines with beyond a teraflop available on them, thanks to the availability of GPUs as an underlying hardware for developing general-purpose applications. We report and show how combining accurate and transferable biophysical VS techniques with these modern massively parallel hardware, allowing significant steps towards more accurate VS screening methods.

Driven by the demand of the game industry, Graphics Processing Units (GPUs) have completed a steady transition from mainframes to workstations to PC cards, where they emerge nowadays like a solid and compelling alternative to traditional computing platforms, delivering extremely high floating point performance and massively parallelism at a very low cost, and thus promoting a new concept of the High Performance Computing (HPC) market; i.e. high performance desktop computing.

This fact has attracted many researchers and encouraged the use of GPUs in a broader range of applications, where developers are required to leverage this technology with new programming models which ease the developer's task of writing programs to run efficiently on GPUs (Garland et al., 2008).

NVIDIA and ATI/AMD, two of the most popular graphics vendors, have released software components which provide simpler access to GPU computing power. CUDA (Compute Unified Device Architecture) (NVIDIA, 2011) is NVIDIA's solution as a simple block-based API for programming; AMD's alternative is called Stream Computing (ATI/AMD, 2011). Those companies have also developed hardware products aimed specifically at the scientific General-Purpose GPU (GPGPU) computing market: Tesla products are from NVIDIA, and Firestream is AMD's product line. More recently (in 2008), the OpenCL[1] framework have emerged as an attempt to unify all of those models with a superset of features, being the first broadly supported multi-platforms data-parallel programming interface for heterogeneous computing, including GPUs and similar devices.

Although these efforts in developing programming models have made great contributions to leverage GPU capabilities, developers have to deal with a massively parallel and throughput-oriented architecture (Garland & Kirk, 2010), which is quite different than traditional computing architectures. Moreover, GPUs are being connected with CPUs through PCI Express bus to build heterogeneous parallel computers, presenting multiple independent memory spaces, a wide spectrum of high speed processing functions, and communication latency between them. These issues drastically increase scaling to a GPU-cluster, bringing additional sources of latency.

Programmability on these platforms is still a challenge, and thus many research efforts have provided abstraction layers avoiding to deal with the hardware particularities of the GPUs and also extracting transparently high level of performance. For example, libraries interfaces for programming with popular programming languages like "Jacket" for Matlab[2],

[1] http://www.khronos.org/opencl/
[2] http://www.accelereyes.com/

or "PyCUDA" or "PyOpenCL" for Python (Klöckner et al., 2011). Some abstraction layers to automatically extract the inherent parallelism existing in many dense linear algebra algorithms, (Agullo et al., 2009), and some of them included as a subroutines in CUDA implementations (Garland et al., 2008; Volkov & Demmel, 2008).

In this review, we give a brief introduction to GPUs in Section 2. Next, we discuss in Section 3 different programming strategies presented in the literature used to overcome the main limitations of VS methods using GPUs, also analyzing their main strengths and weaknesses on single-and-multi GPU-based systems. We also describe in Section 4 our contributions on this field, and finally report our main conclusions about current trends and future predictions in Section5.

2. The roadmap of GPUs as high performance platforms

The graphics hardware has been an active area of research for developing general-purpose computation for many years. The first graphics-oriented machines in which some general purpose applications where developed were the Ikonas (England, 1978), the Pixel Machine (Potmesil & Hoffert, 1989) and Pixel-Planes 5 (Rhoades et al., 1992). These early graphics hardware were typically graphics compute servers rather than desktop workstations.

Moreover, other attempts were made after the wide deployment of GPUs, but still with fixed-function pipelines that were categorized in Trendall & Stewart (2000). For instance, Lengyel et al. (1990) used the rasterization hardware for robot motion planning. Hoff et al. (2001) described the use of z-buffer techniques for the computation of Voronoi diagrams. Kedem & Ishihara (1999) used a graphics hardware to crack the UNIX password encryption. Bohn (1998) also used the graphics hardware in the computation of artificial neural networks. Convolution and wavelet transforms were carried out by Hopf & Ertl (1999), Hopf & Thomas (1999).

However, the milestone to spread GPUs as a general-purpose platform was first motivated by Larsen & McAllister (2001), who demonstrated the capacity of a graphics processor to accelerate a typical dense matrix product through regular texture operators. This result attracted the scientific community into a race for using the GPU as a co-processor, and immediately the number of applications enhanced in that way led to the GPGPU initiative (General-Purpose computation on Graphics Processing Units, also known as GPU Computing and GPGPU.org on the Web) by Mark Harris in 2002 as an attempt to compile all these achievements (Luebke et al., 2006). Soon after, the Cg language was born to ease this path in terms of programmability, trailing earlier achievements like the introduction of fully programmable hardware and an assembly language for specifying programs to run on each vertex (Lindholm et al., 2001) or fragment processors.

GPUs started to be seriously considered in the HPC community mainly due to the raw performance and massively parallelism of GPUs. The programmable shader hardware was explicitly designed to process multiple data-parallel primitives at the same time. Moreover, GPUs typically had multiple vertex and fragment processors. For instance, the NVIDIA GeForce 6800 Ultra had 6 vertex and 16 fragment processors.

Nevertheless, the graphics hardware was very limited for developing general-purpose applications for several reasons that are mainly summarized in two main constraints: (1) hardware constraints and (2) graphics-devoted programming model. On the hardware side, the instruction sets of each processor stage were very limited compared to CPU ones; they were primarily math operations, many of which were graphics-specific and only few control flow operations were available. Moreover, each programmable stage could access constant registers across all primitives and also read-write registers per primitive, but these resources were very limited on their numbers of inputs, outputs, constants, registers and instructions. Fragment processors had the ability to fetch data from textures, so they were capable of memory gather. However, the output address of a fragment was always determined before the fragment was processed -the processor cannot change the output location of a pixel-, so fragment processors were initially not able to do memory scatter. Vertex processors evolved acquiring texture capabilities, and thus they were capable of changing the position of input vertices, which ultimately affect where in the image pixels would be drawn. Therefore, vertex processors became capable of both gather and scatter. Unfortunately, vertex scatter could lead to memory and rasterization coherence issues further down the pipeline. Combined with the lower performance of vertex processors, this limited the utility of vertex scatter in the first generation of current GPUs (Owens et al., 2007).

At the beginning of this new GPGPU era in 2002, the available APIs to interact with the GPUs were DirectX 9 and OpenGL 1.4, both of them designed only to match the features required by the graphics applications. To access the computational resources, programmers had to cast their problems into native graphics operations, thus the only way to launch their computation was through OpenGL or DirectX API calls. For instance, to run many simultaneous instances of a compute function, the computation was written as a pixel shader. The collection of input data was stored in texture images and issued to the GPU by submitting triangles. The output was cast as a set of pixels generated from the raster operations with the hardware constraints previously mentioned (Kirk & Hwu, 2010).

Despite of this worst-case scenario, some applications from different scientific fields were ported to the GPU (Owens et al., 2007) by intrepid researchers. Some early work was presented by Thompson et al. (2002) in which they used the programmable vertex processor of an NVIDIA GeForce 3 GPU to solve the 3-Satisfiability problem and to perform matrix multiplication. Besides, Strzodka showed the multiple 8-bit texture channels combination to create virtual 16-bit floating-point operations (Strzodka, 2002), and Harris analyzed the accumulated error in boiling simulation operations caused by the low precision (Harris, 2002) on early generation of GPUs.

Strzodka constructed and analyzed special discrete schemes which, for certain PDE types, allow reproduction of the qualitative behavior of the continuous solution even with very low computational precision, e.g. 8 bits (Strzodka, 2004).

Other efforts were made in fields such as Physically-Based Simulations, Signal and Image Processing, Segmentation, etc (Owens et al., 2007; Pharr & Fernando, 2005).

With the advent of CUDA from NVIDIA in 2006, programming general-purpose applications on GPUs became more accessible. NVDIA has shipped millions of CUDA-enabled GPUs to date. Software developers, scientists and researchers are finding broad-ranging application fields for CUDA, including image and video processing, computational biology and chemistry, fluid dynamics simulation, CT image reconstruction, seismic analysis, ray tracing and many more (CUD, 2011; Hwu, 2011; Nguyen, 2007; Sanders & Kandrot, 2010).

2.1 GPU computing with CUDA

The increasing popularity and promising results of the *GPGPU* within the field of HPC was leveraged by few intrepid programmers for several reasons: (1) the tough learning curve, particularly for non-graphics experts, (2) the high-potential overhead presented by graphics API, (3) the highly constrained memory layout and access model and (4) the bandwidth requirements of multipass rendering.

The advent of CUDA (Compute Unified Device Architecture) from NVIDIA in November 2006, with a new parallel programming model and instruction set architecture, democratized the *GPGPU* (Luebke, 2007), springing up a new era into the community coined *GPU Computing*. *GPU Computing* means using GPUs for computing through parallel programming language and API; i.e. without using the traditional graphics API and pipeline previously introduced.

CUDA leverages the parallel compute engine in NVIDIA GPUs to solve many complex computational problems without dealing with graphics particularities of the GPU and simply programming in C or C++ with some minimal set of language extensions that are exposed to the programmer. In addition, CUDA comes with a software environment that allows developers to use different high-level programming languages, such as CUDA FORTRAN, OpenCL, DirectCompute[3]. This maintains a low learning curve for programmers familiar with standard programming languages such as C.

CUDA is also a scalable programming model. It is designed to transparently manage tremendous levels of chip-level parallelism through three key abstractions: a hierarchy of thread groups, shared memories and barrier synchronization, providing fine-grained data parallelism and thread parallelism. This scalable programming model has allowed CUDA architecture to span a wide market range by simply scaling the number of processors and memory partitions. NVIDIA provides three different GPU products: GeForce, Quadro and Tesla, which are devoted to different markets (NVIDIA, 2011). The latter is the bet of NVIDIA for the HPC market, enhancing the double-precision performance, increasing the memory partitions, enabling error detection, among others to mention but a few.

2.2 CUDA programming model

The increasing popularity of the CUDA programming model (NVIDIA, 2011) is mainly because it presents two main features previously commented: the scalability and the easy-to-use fact. Next we show how these features are developed in the programming model.

A CUDA program is organized into two different subprograms: *host program* and *device program* or *kernels*. The host program consists of one or more sequential threads running on the CPU (host), which are in charge of initializing, monitoring and finalizing the execution of the device program.

The device program consists of one or more parallel kernels that are suitable for execution on the GPU. A **kernel** executes a scalar sequential program on a set of parallel threads. The programmer organizes these threads into a grid of thread blocks (see Figure 1). A **grid** is composed of several blocks which are equally distributed and scheduled among all multiprocessors on the GPU. A **block** is a batch of threads which can cooperate together

[3] http://developer.nvidia.com/directcompute

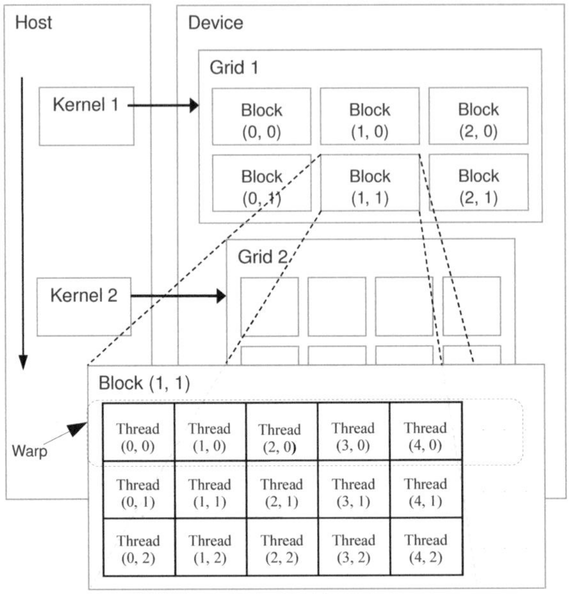

Fig. 1. CUDA programming model

because they are assigned to the same multiprocessor and therefore they share all the resources included in this multiprocessor, such as register file and a high-speed, per-block on-chip memory (called *shared memory*) for inter-thread communication. They are also allowed to synchronize with each other via barriers. Threads from different blocks in the same grid can only coordinate via operations in a shared global memory space (called *device memory*) visible to all threads. The **thread** is the basic execution unit that is mapped to a single core (called *Stream Processor*). Finally, threads included in a block are divided into batches of 32 threads called **warps**. The warp is the scheduled unit, so the threads of the same block are scheduled in a given multiprocessor warp by warp. The programmer declares the number of blocks, the number of threads per block and their distribution to arrange parallelism given the program constraints (i.e., data and control dependencies).

The CUDA programming model presents several patterns of parallelism depending on the previous thread hierarchy. For instance, all threads in a warp execute at the same time the same instruction over different data in a SIMD fashion. However, CUDA requires that thread blocks are independent, meaning that a kernel must execute correctly no matter the order in which blocks are run. Therefore, different thread blocks execute different instructions at a given time, which fit better in a MIMD fashion. This MIMD pattern is one of the key issues in the CUDA programming model as it is the way to ensure scalability, but it also implies that the need for global communication or synchronization amongst threads is the main consideration when it comes to decompose parallel work into separate kernels (Garland et al., 2008).

3. Virtual screening methods on GPUs

In this Section, we summarize the main technical contributions for the parallelization of VS methods on GPUs available on the bibliography. Concretely, we pay special attention to the parallelization of docking methods on GPUs.

In terms of implementations, the trend seems to be reusing available libraries when possible and implement the achievements into existing simulation packages for VS. Among the most-used strategies are either implementing the most time-consuming parts of previously designed codes for serial computers, or redesigning the whole code from scratch. When porting VS methods to GPUs, we should realize that not all methods are equally amenable for optimization. Programmers should check carefully how the code works and whether it is suited for the target architecture. Irrespective of CUDA, most authors maintain that the application will be more accessible in the future thanks to new and promising programming paradigms which are still in the experimental stage or are not yet broadly used. Among them, we may highlight OpenCL or DirectCompute.

3.1 Dock6.2

Yang et al. (2010) present a GPU accelerated amber score in Dock6.2 [4]. They report up to 6.5x speedup factor with respect to 3,000 cycles during MD simulation compared to a dual core CPU. The lack of the single-precision floating point operations in the targeted GPU (NVIDIA GeForce 9800GT) produces small precision losses compared to the CPU, which the authors assume as acceptable. They highlight the thread management utilizing multiple blocks and single transferring of the molecule grids as the main factor that dominates the performance improvements on GPU. They use another optimization techniques, such as dealing with the latency attributed to thread synchronization, divergence hidden and shared memory through tiling, that authors state may double the speedup of the MD simulation. We miss a deeper analysis on the device memory bandwidth utilization. It is not clear whether the pattern accesses to device memory in the different versions of the designs presented here are coalesced or not, which may drastically affect the overall performance.

They finally conclude that the speedup of Amber scoring is limited by the Amdahl's law for two main reasons: (1) the rest of the Amber scoring takes a higher percentage of the run time than the portion parallelized on the GPU, and (2) Partitioning the work among SMs will eventually decrease the individual job size to a point where the overhead of initializing an SP dominates the application execution time. However, we do not see any clear evaluation that supports these conclusions.

3.2 Autodock

Kannan & Ganji (2010) migrate part of a molecular docking application, *Autodock* to NVIDIA GPUs. Concretely, they only focus on the Genetic Algorithm (GA) which is used to find the optimal docking position of a ligand to a protein. They use single-precision floating point operation arguing that, "GA depends on relative goodness among individual energies and single precision may not affect the accuracy of GA path significantly". All the data relative to the GA state is maintained on the GPU memory, avoiding data movement through the PCI Express bus.

The GA algorithms need random numbers for the selection process. They decide to generate the random numbers on the CPU instead of doing on the GPU. The explanation of that is two-fold according to the authors: (1) It enables one to one comparisons of CPU and GPU results, and (2) it reduces the design, coding and validation effort of generating random

[4] http://dock.compbio.ucsf.edu/DOCK_6/

numbers on GPU. From our point of view this decision contradicts the previous assumption of maintaining the data on the GPU, and we do not see enough arguments on these two sentences.

A very nice decision is what the authors call *CGPU Memory Manager* that enables alignment for individual memory request, support for pinned memory and join memory transfer to do all of them in just one transfer. Regarding the fitness function of the GA, authors decide to evaluate all the individuals in a population regardless of modifications. This avoids warp divergences although it makes some redundant work.

Three different parallel design alternatives are discussed in this regard. Two of them only differ in the way they calculate the fitness function, assigning the calculation of the fitness of an individual either to a GPU thread or GPU block. A good comparison between them is provided. The last one includes an extra management of the memory to avoid atomic operations which drastically penalizes the performance.

All of these implementations are rewarded with up to 50x in the fitness calculation but they do not mention anything about global speedup of the Autodock program.

3.3 FFT-based rigid docking

Feng et al. (2010) use a FFT-based method to predict rigid docking configurations, achieving up to 3x speedup factor with its sequential counterpart version. However, FFT is not well suited to be implemented on GPUs, as long as more computations are not being developed afterwards. Moreover, the best implementation of FFT on GPUs (Volkov & Kazian, 2008) up to now is not referenced in this paper. Therefore, it is not clear whether the authors have overcome this implementation or not, and the real benefits of taking this approach for docking.

3.4 Multiple GPU docking

Roh et al. (2009) propose the parallelization of a molecular docking system on GPUs. They obtain 33 to 287 speedups for the calculation of electrostatics and van der Waals energies using different strategies and scaling the number of GPUs until reach two GPUs. Finally, global speedups of up to 2 times are achieved compared to a sequential counterpart version. However, they do not show any practical application of their code. They highlight that an efficient strategy to leverage the power of multiple GPU system is necessary. They also report the importance of an efficient visualization method.

3.5 Genetic algorithms based docking

Korb et al. (2011) enhance the PLANTS (Korb et al., 2006) approach for protein-ligand docking using GPUs. They report speedup factors of up to 50x in their GPU implementation compared to an optimized CPU based implementation for the evaluation of interaction potentials in the context of rigid protein. The GPU implementation was carried out using OpenGL to access the GPU's pipeline and Nvidia's Cg language for implementing the shaders programs (i.e. Cg kernels to compute on the GPU). Using this way of programming GPUs, the programming effort is too high, and also some peculiarities of the GPU architecture may be limited. For instance, the authors say that some of the spatial data structures used in the CPU implementation can not directly be mapped to the GPU programming model because of missing support for shared memory operations (Korb et al., 2011).

The speedup factors observed, especially for small ligands, are limited by several factors. First, only the ligand and protein conformation generation and scoring function evaluation are carried out on the GPU whereas the optimization algorithm is run on the CPU. This algorithmic decomposition implies time-consuming data transfers through PCI Express bus. The optimization algorithm used in PLANTS is the Ant Colony Optimization (ACO) algorithm (Dorigo, 1992). Concretely, authors propose a parallel scheme for this algorithm on a CPU cluster, which use multiple ant colonies in parallel, exchanging information occasionally between them (Manfrin et al., 2006). Developing the ACO algorithm on the GPU as it has been shown in Cecilia et al. (2011) can drastically reduce the communications overhead between CPU and GPU.

3.6 Binding site mapping

Another key point in docking applications is the prediction or estimation of regions on a protein surface that are likely to bind a small molecule with high affinity.

Sukhwani & Herbordt (2010) present a fast, GPU-based implementation of FTMap, a production binding site mapping program. Both the rigid-docking and the energy minimization phases are accelerated, resulting in a 13x overall speedup of the entire application over the current single-core implementation. While an efficient multicore implementation of FTMap may be possible, it is certainly challenging: they estimate it would require an effort greater than what they have spent on the GPU mapping.

The first step assumes the interacting molecules to be rigid and performs exhaustive 3D search to find the best pocket on the protein that can fit the probe. This step is called rigid docking. The top scoring conformations from this step are saved for further evaluation in the second step. The second step models the flexibility in the side chains of the probes by allowing them to move freely and minimizing the energy between the protein-probe complex.

Overall, this work provides a cost-effective, desktop-based alternative to the large clusters currently being used by production mapping servers. Essential to the success of this work is restructuring the original application in several places, e.g., to avoid the use of neighbor lists.

In the future, they plan on extending this work to a multi-GPU implementation and integrating it into a production web server.

4. Testimonials of porting docking algorithm on GPUs

In this Section, we introduce different success stories of porting docking algorithms to GPUs that we have worked on. We also contribute with some novelties in this field; we have worked in this direction and focused on the parallel implementation, incorporation of new improvements in the underlying VS methodology, and exploitation of the docking program FlexScreen which its sequential version is described in Section 4.1. The different strategies we have followed to tame GPUs for FlexScreen can be also used in any VS method.

In Sections 4.2, 4.3 and 4.4, we describe different approaches we have followed for the acceleration of the calculation of non-bonded interactions. In Figure 2 we can see an overview of the main results obtained for the parallelization of the electrostatics kernel using a full coulomb approach (direct summation) or a grid one. In Section 4.5 we show the implementation of a kernel for the fast calculation of SASA (Solvent Accessible Surface Area), widely used in implicit solvation models.

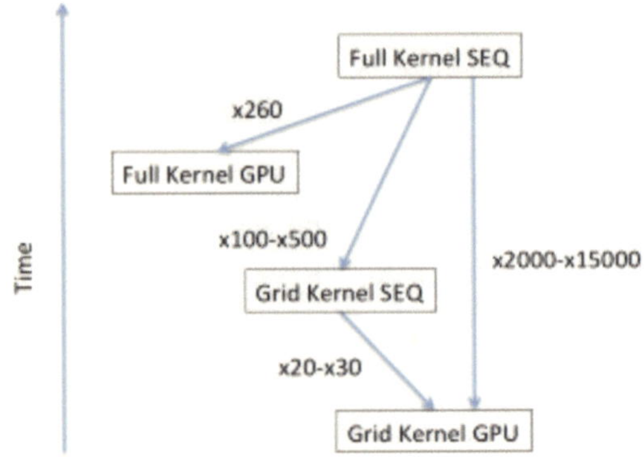

Fig. 2. Comparative of the accelerations obtained using the different kernels in their SEQ (Sequential) and GPU versions for the electrostatics calculation

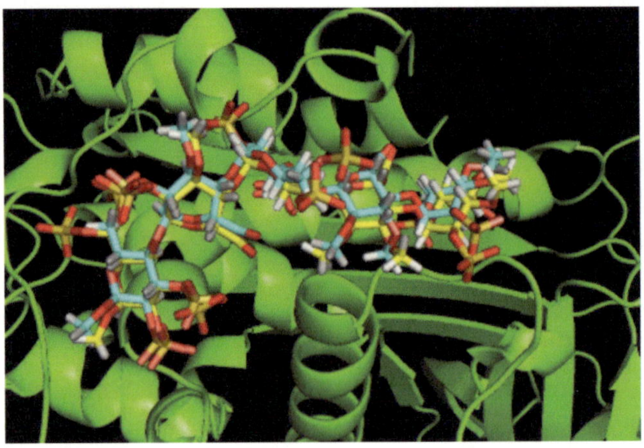

Fig. 3. FlexScreen docking prediction for the binding pose of Heparin with Antithrombin. The model for heparin contains up to 200 atoms and 20 rotatable bonds. Experimental binding pose is yellow colored while FlexScreen prediction is blue colored. Root mean square deviation is less than 1 Å

4.1 Docking with FlexScreen

FlexScreen (Merlitz et al., 2004) performs receptor–ligand docking simulations using an atomistic representation of the protein and the ligand. Ligands are docked using a cascaded version (Fischer et al., 2007) of a stochastic tunneling algorithm (Merlitz et al., 2003) which samples translations of the center-of-mass and rotations of the ligand, as well as intra-molecular conformational changes. In addition to the degrees of freedom of the ligand, receptor conformational change is accounted for in selected side chains. An optimized docked conformation is shown in Figure 3. Previous work demonstrated that this approach yields accurate results for binding mode prediction and improves selectivity in library screens for a number of pharmaceutically relevant receptors (Kokh & Wenzel, 2008).

The FlexScreen scoring function is based on adaptable biophysical models, including electrostatic, Van der Waals, hydrogen bonds and a solvation contribution. For the calculation of electrostatic and Van der Waals terms during the docking simulation, precomputed grids that represent the protein are used (Meng et al., 1992). FlexScreen is divided into two programs; *dogrid,* which performs the electrostatic (ES) and Van der Waals (VDW) precalculation in form of a grid for a given receptor structure and *dock,* which reads the previously generated ES and VDW grid files and carries out the docking simulation for a single ligand or ligand database.

4.2 Full calculation of the non-bonded interactions

In this section, we focus on the optimization of the full version (direct summation) of the calculation of non-bonded interactions (such as electrostatics and van der Waals forces), as this kernel is an important bottleneck to different VS methods (Perez Sanchez & Wenzel, 2011). On GPUs, Stone et al. (Stone et al., 2007) reached speedups of around 100 times, while Harvey et al. (Harvey & De Fabritiis, 2009) achieve a 200 times acceleration. We test our kernel in GPUs to exploits the parallelism of this application, getting up to 260 times speedup compared to its sequential version.

Algorithm 1 Sequential pseudocode for the calculation of electrostatic interactions for a receptor ligand case, full kernel version (direct summation)

```
for i = 0 to nrec do
    for j = 0 to nlig do
        calculus(rec[i], lig[j])
    end for
end for
```

In order to exploit all the resources available on the GPU, and get the maximum benefit from CUDA, we focus first on finding ways to parallelise the sequential version of the electrostatic interaction kernel, which is shown in Algorithm 1, where *rec* is the biggest molecule, *lig* the smallest molecule, *nrec* the number of atoms of *rec* and *nlig* the number of atoms of *lig*.

In our approach, CUDA threads are in charge of calculating the interaction between atoms. However, the task developed by the CUDA thread blocks in this application can drastically affect the overall performance. To avoid communication overheads, each thread block should contain all the information related to the ligand or protein. Two alternatives come along to get this. The former is to identify each thread block with information about the biggest molecule; i.e. CUDA threads are overloaded, and there are few thread blocks running in parallel. The latter is exactly the opposite, to identify each thread as one atom of that molecule and then CUDA threads are light-weight, and there are many thread blocks ready for execution. The second alternative fits better in the GPU architecture idiosyncrasy.

Figure 4 shows this design. Each atom from the biggest molecule is represented by a single thread. Then, every CUDA thread goes through all the atoms of the smallest molecule.

Algorithm 2 outlines the GPU pseudocode we have implemented. Notice that, before and after the kernel call, it is needed to move the data between the CPU RAM and the GPU memory.

The kernel implementation is straightforward from Figure 4. Each thread simply performs the electrostatic interaction calculations with its corresponding atom of the *rec* molecule and all the *lig* molecule atoms.

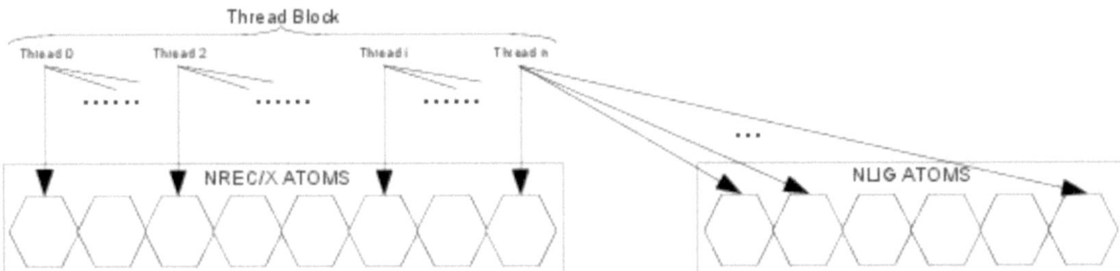

Fig. 4. GPU design for X thread blocks (with $X = 1$) with n threads layout.

Algorithm 2 GPU pseudocode for the full ES kernel.

$CopyDataFromCPUtoGPU(rec)$
$CopyDataFromCPUtoGPU(lig)$
$numBlocks := nrec/numThreads$
Kernel$(numBlocks, numThreads)$
$CopyDataFromGPUtoCPU(result)$

CUDA Kernels

Algorithm 3. Basic implementation

for all Blocks **do**
  for $i = 0$ to $nlig$ **do**
    $calculus(myAtomRec, lig[i])$
  end for
end for

Algorithm 4. Tiles implementation

for all Blocks **do**
  $numIt = nlig/numThreads$
  for $i = 0$ to $numIt$ **do**
    $copyBlockDataToSharedMemory(lig)$
    $calculusBlock(myAtomRec, ligBlock)$
  end for
end for

We have derived two different implementations: the basic one (Algorithm 3), and the advanced one (Algorithm 4), where a blocking (or tiling) technique is applied to increase the performance of the application, grouping atoms of the *lig* molecule in blocks and taking them to the *shared memory*, taking advantage in this way of the very low access latency to the *shared memory*.

4.2.1 Performance evaluation

The performance of our sequential and GPU implementations are evaluated in a quad-core Intel Xeon E5530 (Nehalem with 8 MB L2 cache), which acts as a host machine for our NVIDIA Tesla C1060 GPU. We compare it with a Cell implementation (Pérez-Sánchez, 2009) in a IBM BladeCenter QS21 with 16 SPE.

Figure 5 shows the execution times for all our implementations (both GPU and Cell) taking into account the data transfer between the RAM memory and the corresponding device memory. All the calculations are performed in simple precision floating point, due the smaller number of double precision units of the Tesla C1060. The benchmarks are executed by varying the number of atoms of the smallest molecule and also the number of atoms of the biggest molecule for studying the cases of protein-protein and ligand-protein interactions. In Figure

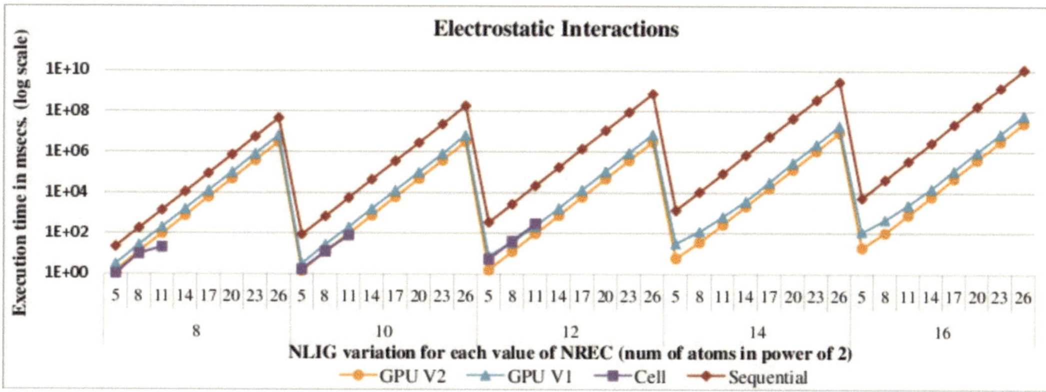

Fig. 5. Results obtained for different molecular size ratios. The execution time for the calculation of the electrostatic potential, in single precision, executed 128 times in a loop for different conformations of the molecule.

5 the performance of the Cell implementation, GPU basic implementation (GPU V1) and GPU tiles implementation (GPU V2) enhances along with the value of *nrec*, defeating the sequential code by a wide margin (up to a speed factor of 260x). Notice that, the speedup factor between GPU and CPU increases faster when the value of *nrec* is higher. It is because the number of thread blocks running in parallel is also higher, and then the GPU resources are fully used. Similarly, for larger values of *nlig*, the speedup factor between GPU and CPU increases also because there are more threads running at the same time. However, it remains flat for a configuration greater than 256 threads per block.

Cell processor is not able to execute some of the biggest benchmarks due to its hardware constraints, mainly related to the 256K SPE Local Storage. However, it performs similarly well compared to the GPUs for the smallest benchmarks in which the GPU is not fully used.

The results obtained for GPU are indeed promising, given the obtained speedup values up to 260x, compared to its sequential version. Cell processor gives similar results to GPUs only in some cases, where the molecules are small and the saturation situation for the GPU is not reached, but for higher workloads GPUs attain speedup values 7 times higher than the Cell processor. This way we can work with bigger molecules and thus perform more realistic calculations.

4.3 Precomputation of grids

In the recent years, the completion of the human genome project has brought new and still unprocessed information about potential targets for the treatment of human diseases with drugs. It is well known that the efficacy of a drug can be vastly improved through the interaction with multiple targets, although undesirable side effects must also be studied. Therefore, it is very important to identify and validate all potential targets for a given compound. Experimental approaches for this purpose are very expensive and time consuming, while in-silico approaches like Virtual Screening (VS) can efficiently propose accurate predictions that drastically reduce testing procedures in the laboratory.

Multiple target drug screening is a particular case of VS methods. In the approach that we propose, the main bottleneck of the calculations is related with the computation of non-bonded kernels in a specific way, concretely the precomputation of potential grids. We show in this Section its acceleration by means of GPUs.

From the other side, VS approaches for multiple target identification have not been yet fully explored. Docking methods have been traditionally applied to ligand database screening (Yuriev et al., 2011), where a large ligand database is screened against a single receptor molecule in order to predict potential leads. The inverse approach, the one we are interested in, where a large database of target receptors is screened against a single ligand, has not received such attention and only some attempts are reported (Hui-fang et al., 2010). In both application scenarios, most docking programs represent the receptor as a rigid molecule (Yuriev et al., 2011) thus limiting the range of applicability of their predictions. There are few reported cases where receptor flexibility has been successfully used in docking simulations (Kokh et al., 2011), but it is clear its relevance and importance for multi target drug screening.

For a realistic simulation of one receptor-ligand pair in *FlexScreen* (Section 4.1) it takes around 80% of the total running time for *dogrid* and 20% for *dock*. In the application case of multiple target drug screening we need to screen one ligand against a large database of receptors, therefore the main bottleneck is the generation of grids by *dogrid*. Even more, ES and VDW grids generated by *dogrid* can also be used for protein surface screening or blind docking (Hetényi & van der Spoel, 2002), an approach where no assumption is done about the part of the receptor where the docking starts. In this situation, we need to determine it first, and the fast examination of ES and VDW grids yields valuable information about potential binding sites, as it has already been shown for the discovery of inhibitors for antithrombin (Meliciani et al., 2009; Navarro-Fernandez et al., 2010). Therefore, our main interest in order to achieve an optimized implementation of multiple target drug screening with flexible receptors is to target our efforts to the acceleration of *dogrid*.

4.3.1 Code design

In this part, we introduce several different GPU designs for the generation of the electrostatic (ES) and Van der (VDW) Waals grids. Firstly, the CPU baselines of that generation are presented before introducing the GPU design proposal. Calculations are always carried out in double precision floating point.

4.3.1.1 Grid calculation on the CPU

In the sequential version of FlexScreen, precomputation of electrostatic (ES) and Van der (VDW) Waals grids is performed in the *dogrid* program as follows; the protein is placed inside a cube of minimal volume $Vol = L^3$ that encloses the protein. A three dimensional grid is created dividing the cube into $(N-1)^3$ smaller cubes of identical volume, each one of side length $d = L/N$, so that the total number of grid points is N^3.

$$V_{elec,i} = \sum_{j=1}^{NREC} \frac{q_j}{r_{ij}} \tag{1}$$

The electrostatic potential due to all protein atoms is calculated on each grid point i according to the Coulomb expression given by equation 1. The total number of atoms of the protein is equal to $NREC$, while q_i is the charge of each individual atom i of the receptor and r_{ij} the distance between point i of the grid and atom j of the receptor. This information is represented

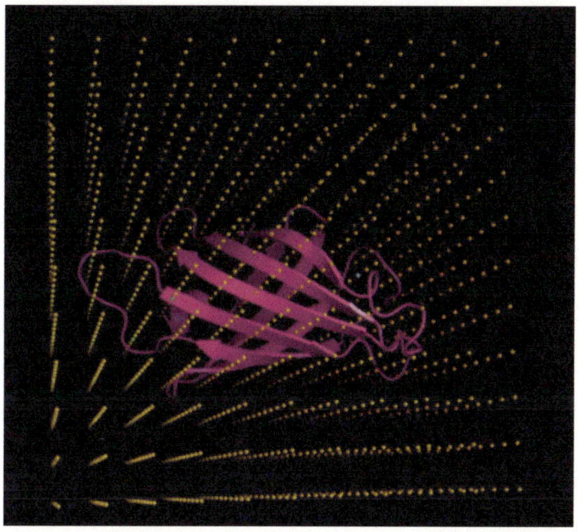

Fig. 6. Grid for streptavidin. Length of the side of the cube (L) is 50 Å, spacing between grid points (d is 5 Å, and the total number of grid points is equal to 11^3

Algorithm 5 Sequential pseudocode for ES grid

for $i_x = 1$ to N **do**
  for $i_y = 1$ to N **do**
    for $i_z = 1$ to N **do**
      for $j = 1$ to $NREC$ **do**
        $calculus(rec[j], ESgrid[i_x, i_y, i_z])$
      end for
    end for
  end for
end for

by *rec*[*j*] for all receptor atoms. The pseudocode is shown in Algorithm 5, where *calculus* performs the calculation of the electrostatic potential following equation 1 for each grid point (defined by its grid indexes i_x, i_y and i_z) computing the non-bonded interactions against all protein atoms and storing conveniently the values in the ES grid file.

$$V_{vdw,i} = 4\epsilon_{ij} \sum_{j=1}^{NREC} \left[\left(\frac{\sigma_{ij}}{r_{ij}} \right)^{12} - \left(\frac{\sigma_{ij}}{r_{ij}} \right)^{6} \right] \quad (2)$$

The calculation of the VDW potential in the *dock* program is performed following equation 2 where ϵ_{ij} and σ_{ij} are the VDW OPLS force field parameters (Jorgensen, 1996) that depend on the type of interacting atoms. Given the fact that the VDW potential decays very fast at short distances, it is convenient to define a cutoff radius r_{cutoff}. Then, we calculate in the scoring funcion the VDW potential only in the cases where atoms are closer than this distance, since for larger values it is very close to zero. Avoiding calculation in those cases we can speed up the global VDW computation. The default r_{cutoff} value used is 4 Å. For this purpose the VDW grid is precalulated in *dogrid*, and it contains on each VDW grid point only information about the indexes of all protein atoms that fulfill this distance condition around each grid

Algorithm 6 Sequential pseudocode for VDW grid

```
for i_x = 1 to N do
  for i_y = 1 to N do
    for i_z = 1 to N do
      for j = 1 to NREC do
        if isNeighbour(i_x, i_y, i_z, rec[j]) then
          store(VDWgrid[i_x, i_y, i_z], j)
        end if
      end for
      sort(VDWgrid[i_x, i_y, i_z], MAXNB)
    end for
  end for
end for
```

point. As shown in Algorithm 6, once r_{cutoff} is defined, for each grid point (i_x, i_y, i_z) we check individually against all the NREC receptor atoms which of them are closer than this distance. Once this check is finished, we sort them and store only the closest $MAXNB$ neighbouring atoms. We have previously tested that a value of 20 for $MAXNB$ yields accurate results for VDW energies.

4.3.1.2 Grid calculation on GPU

We describe in this part the strategy we followed for the calculation of the ES and VDW grids on the GPU.

Algorithm 7 GPU pseudocode for Electrostatic (ES) grid

Host (CPU)

```
CopyDataCPUtoGPU(rec)
nBlocks := ngp/numThreads * NREC/AT_BLOCK
Kernel <<< nBlocks, numThreads >>> (rec, ESGrid)
CopyDataFromGPUtoCPU(ESGrid)
```

Device (GPU)

```
for all nBlocks do
  copyBlockDataToSM(rec, AT_BLOCK)
  for i = 0 to AT_BLOCK do
    calculus(energy, rec[i])
  end for
  atomicAdd(&ESGrid[myCell], energy)
end for
```

Algorithm 7 describes the calculation of the Electrostatic (ES) grid on GPU. Firstly, all information related to the receptor (atomic positions and partial charges) and represented by *rec* in the pseudocode is copied from CPU's host memory to GPU's device memory. Moreover, the ES grid is allocated on device memory.

The ES grid is divided into thread-blocks, having as many thread-blocks as the total number of grid points ($ngp = N^3$) divided by the number of threads ($numThreads$), which is actually a degree of freedom. Moreover, per each of these thread-blocks, we set $NREC/AT\_BLOCK$ thread-blocks, being AT_BLOCK (number of atoms per block) a fixed value which is a degree of freedom as well.

All threads in a thread-block collaborate to obtain a coalesced access to device memory, and also to prepare a tiling technique. The former is guaranteed as threads in the same warp access to the same memory segment. Moreover, the tiling technique is implemented; .initially all threads collaborate to store in shared memory (SM) the information pertaining to its block of protein atoms, i.e. *AT_BLOCK* and afterwards the *calculus* function is performed for a given point of the ES grid, represented by i_x, i_y, i_z. Finally the result is stored back in the ES grid.

It should be noticed that the same data-block from *rec* is loaded as many times as thread-blocks represent the ES grid; i.e. $ngp/numThreads$, but this is done by different thread-blocks. Finally, atomic operations are performed to sum up individual values calculated by the different threads. ES grid data is copied back to host memory and written to disk.

Algorithm 8 GPU pseudocode for Van der Waals (VDW) grid

Host (CPU)

```
CopyDataFromCPUtoGPU(rec)
nBlocks := ngp
KernelVDW <<< nBlocks, numThreads >>> (rec, VDWGrid)
CopyDataFromGPUtoCPU(VDWGrid)
```

Device (GPU)

```
for all ngp do
    for i = 0 to 1NREC/numThreads
    do
        StoreInSM(neighbourhoodShared, i, isNeighbour(i, rec[i], r_cutoff))
    end for
    if tid == 0and numNeighbours > MAXNB then
        sort(neighbourhoodShared)
    end if
    VDWGrid[i_x, i_y, i_z] = neighbourhoodShared
end for
```

The calculation of the Van der Waals (VDW) grid on the GPU is described by Algorithm 8. Each thread-block calculates neighbours for each grid point of the VDW grid. Moreover, the *rec* information (atoms of the receptor) is equally divided into threads of each thread-block, assigning different sets of *rec* to each thread. Thus each thread calculates the distance between the grid point (represented by i_x, i_y, i_z) of its thread-block and all atoms in the *rec* set associated with it.

For those atoms closer than cutoff radius r_{cutoff}, threads store their indexes and distance values in an array represented by *neighbourhoodShared*. This process is performed in shared memory to avoid costly accesses to device memory. If the number of neighbours found for a given cell is bigger than the maximum number of neighbour ($MAXNB$), they are sorted and only the $MAXNB$ closest-neighbours are stored as final result for the VDW grid. Finally VDW grid data is copied back to host memory and written to disk.

4.3.2 Performance evaluation

In what follows our hardware platforms are: (1) a dual-socket 2.40 GHz quad-core Intel Xeon E5620 Westmere(R) processor, and (2) a NVIDIA Geforce GTX 465 based on Fermi architecture released in November 2010 (NVIDIA, 2009). We use GNU *gcc* version 4.3.4 with the -O3 flag to compile our CPU implementations, and CUDA compilation tools (release 4.0) on the GPU side.

The code of *dogrid* was profiled using the GNU tool *gprof* (Graham et al., 2004) and by manual introduction of timers in the code, yielding similar results in both cases for different protein sizes and grid densities (represented by N^3). It is desirable to use as many grid points

ngp	Ex. time (CPU)	GFLOPS (CPU)	% Ex. time ES (CPU)	% Ex. time ES (GPU)	Speedup ES	Speedup VDW	Global Speedup	GFLOPS ES	GFLOPS VDW	TOTAL GFLOPS
17^3	171.637	0.764	90.7	33.4	131.26	6.74	48.42	62.64	30.94	37.2
33^3	1372.59	0.77	90.67	27.24	155.09	5.97	46.6	74.04	27.22	37.7
65^3	10908.779	0.77	91.2	31.97	160.2	7.27	56.17	76.5	35.3	46.2
129^3	86950.656	0.78	91.7	35.8	163.13	8.27	63.7	77.1	42.26	52.96
193^3	290558.25	0.77	91.7	36.9	159.5	8.45	64.2	76.2	43.7	54.34

Table 1. Results obtained for different grid densities (specified by ngp, number of grid points) for the protein streptavidin (1740 atoms) in a cubic grid of volume 32^3 Å^3. Ex. time means execution time in milliseconds.

as possible for the grid, since interpolation strategies are used later in the *dock* program to calculate the Van der Waals and electrostatic energies in the scoring function. Higher number of grid points imply smaller spacing between grid points and therefore more accuracy for the interpolation procedure. However, the size of the grid grows with N^3 and consequently the necessary memory storage also increases. Nevertheless, we have found that a satisfactory approach consists in the use of already tested average grid spacing values that yield good accuracy in the docking calculations. We have tested it and found that a grid spacing value of 0.5 Å gives a good compromise between accuracy and memory requirements. In these cases, ES grid calculation takes around 80 % of the *dogrid* running time while the calculation of the VDW grid takes around 20 %. Less than 1 % of the time is involved in input file reads and final grid file writes. According to Amdahl's law (Amdahl, 1967) it is clear that if we focus on individual acceleration of both ES and VDW grid calculations and succeed, global *dogrid* program would achieve high speedups.

We summarize in this part the main results obtained in our GPU implementation.

Table 1 shows different performance parameters obtained with our CPU (*dogrid* program) and GPU versions of the ES and VDW grid calculations for the protein streptavidin. In the different columns, we specify the total number of grid points used in the grid, the percentage of time spent in the ES grid computations (for VDW grid it can be inferred substracting it from 100 %) in both CPU and GPU versions, the speed-up factor obtained by the GPU grid calculations of ES and VDW grids compared to the sequential counterpart version, and finally the maximum values of GFLOPS obtained by our GPU codes. It is noteworthy to remark that we count the *sqrt* and *mad* operations as a single and double FLOP respectively. When the number of grid points increases, performance of the sequential version remains constant, while the performance of the GPU implementation slightly increases reaching saturation values.

The maximum speed-up factor attained by the ES grid calculation for streptavidin reaches 163x, while for the VDW grid calculation we report a maximal 8x speed-up factor. The lower speedup value obtained for the latter kernel is due to the less arithmetic-intensity kernel and to a higher number of synchronization constraints than in the former. Global speedups for *dogrid* attain accelerations in the $50 - 60$ speedup range. It is also worth mentioning that the calculations have been performed in double precision. We have checked that switching from double to single precision in the Fermi GPU changes ES grid speedup factor from 160 to 250 times. Since same memory can be now filled with two times more protein information, less time is involved in data transfer and more in computations in single floating point arithmetic, which is faster than for double precision, both factors contributing to the higher speedup. Nevertheless, we decided to work always in double precision for the grid generation, given the required accuracy for the docking simulations.

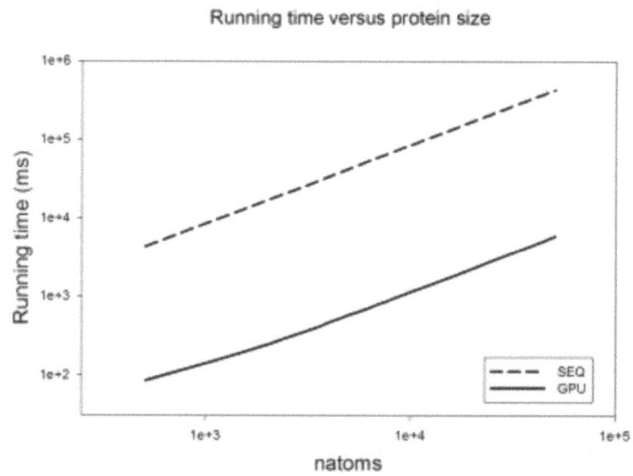

Fig. 7. Running times in miliseconds for the ES and VDW grid calculations obtained with the sequential version (dashed line) and GeForce GTX 465 GPU version (continous line) versus the total number of atoms (natoms) taken from the protein. Both axes are in logarithmic scale. Protein chosen is mammalian fatty acid synthase (PDB ID: 2UVZ)

In order to measure the performance of our parallel implementation we calculated the number of floating point operation per seconds, specified in terms of GFLOPS, for double precision. For the best cases we have obtained a maximum of 77 and 43 GFLOPS for both ES and VDW grid implementation, which is translated into a global 53 GFLOPS performance measure for the whole program, clearly outperforming the performance of 0.7 GFLOPS obtained by the sequential version. Nevertheless, we think that there is still room for improvement in our implementation, concretely for the VDW grid GPU kernel.

Previous results from Table 1 have been obtained for streptavidin, medium-small size protein, but we have checked that for bigger proteins and the global acceleration results remain in the same range. Regarding applicability range of our implementation, the usual protein sizes involved in drug screening tend to be between 1000 to 100000 atoms. We have studied how does our implementation behave in this range of receptor sizes. In Figure 7, we mesaure total running time for the generation of ES and VDW grids for both the sequential and GPU (GeForce GTX 465) implementations. We have chosen mammalian fatty acid synthase as study protein since with 60000 atoms it is one of the biggest proteins feasible for docking calculations. We have performed our calculations varying the number of atoms used in the grid computations. It can be clearly seen that a two orders of magnitude speedup is obtained for the GPU implementation over the whole protein size range, so we are sure that our implementation is valid in a long protein size range as happen usually in multi target drug screening calculations.

In this Section, we have efficiently shown how the CUDA language can be used to exploit the GPU architecture in an applied drug discovery problem. At this point and as far as we know, this is the first GPU implementation of a multiple target drug screening methodology.

We have accelerated the grid generation of the docking program FlexScren for multiple target drug screening using the CUDA language for the GPU architecture. We have obtained average speedups of up to 160 and 8 times for the acceleration of ES and VDW grid calculations for a

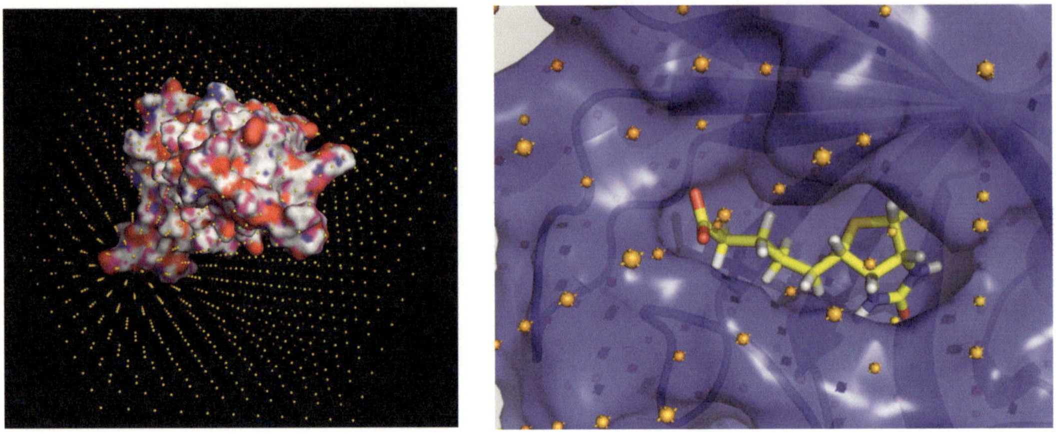

Fig. 8. (A) Representation of the grid for the protein streptavidin. Length of the side of the cube (L) is 50 Å, spacing between grid points d is 5 Å, and the total number of grid points is equal to 11^3. (B) Biotin in the binding pocket of streptavidin

range of proteins in the 1000 − 10000 atoms size range with high accuracy in double floating point precision. These are translated to global speedups of up to 60 times for the program *dogrid*.

4.4 Calculation of non-bonded interactions using grids

We have described in Section 4.2 how the bottleneck of VS methods are related with the computation of full non-bonded interactions Kernels and how GPUs can yield speedups of up to 260 times (Guerrero et al., 2011). Nevertheless, mentioned Kernels need to perform N^2 interactions calculations (N = total number of particles in the system) and even using GPUs, the required computation time grows polynomically with N so this imposes serious limitations for the simulation of big size systems. Thus we decided to look for alternatives to full Kernels and decided to use grid Kernels (Meng et al., 1992). We have checked that just in the sequential version, speedups of 200 times versus the full non-bonded Kernel are obtained. In Section 4.3 we have reported how the calculation of the grids is performed.

We describe in this Section how to unleash the potential of GPUs for the calculation of non-bonded potentials in VS using grids. Previous works have investigated this approach in a similar fashion but for long range interactions using Ewald-Mesh methods (Cerutti et al., 2009). Given the molecular sizes involved in protein-ligand interactions, we are only interested in short-range electrostatics. Related works reported a 3 times speedup using a different approach (Feng et al., 2010), a 50 times speedup focusing on the acceleration of more particular Kernels of the docking program Autodock (Kannan & Ganji, 2010), and a 7 times acceleration of the Dock6 scoring function by Yang et al. (2010).

The protein is placed inside a cube of minimal volume $Vol = L^3$ that encloses it. A three dimensional grid is created dividing the cube into $(N-1)^3$ smaller cubes of identical volume, each one of side length $d = L/N$, so that the total number of grid points is N^3. The electrostatic potential due to all protein atoms is calculated on each grid point i according to the Coulomb expression (Meng et al., 1992). A graphical depiction of the grid for streptavidin can be seen in Figure 8(A), and in more detail for the ligand biotin on its binding pocket in Figure 8(B).

Once the protein grid is loaded into memory, the calculation of the electrostatic potential for the protein-ligand system is performed as follows: for each ligand atom i with charge q_i at point P_i we calculate which are the eight closest protein grid point neighbours. Next, an interpolation procedure is applied to estimate the value of the electrostatic potential due to all protein atoms at P_i. The same procedure is applied to all ligand atoms summing them up. Different interpolation procedures in 3D have been used (Press et al., 1992); linear, cubic and Gauss interpolation.

4.4.1 Code design

In this Section, we introduce the CPU and GPU designs for the calculation of the electrostatic (ES) potential using grids. We have used NVIDIA's CUDA (NVIDIA, 2010) for the GPU implementations on two different machines; a) a host Intel Xeon E6850 CPU with a NVIDIA GeForce GTX 465 GPU and b) a host Intel Xeon E5620 with a NVIDIA Tesla C2050 GPU. They are referred to as Fermi and Tesla. We use GNU *gcc* version 4.3.4 with the -O3 flag to compile our CPU implementations, and CUDA compilation tools (release 4.0) on the GPU side.

4.4.1.1 ES energy calculation on CPU

Algorithm 9 Sequential pseudocode for the calculation of the electrostatic potential

```
for i = 1 to N do
    for j = 1 to nlig do
        energy[i * nlig + j] =
        interpolate(lig[i * nlig + j], ESGrid)
    end for
end for
```

We perform a VS experiment where a ligand database containing up to thousands of ligands is screened against a single protein molecule. The precomputed protein grid is read from file and loaded onto memory. Next, the electrostatic (ES) energy of each atom is calculated using interpolation on the grid as explained before and following the pseudocode shown in Algorithm 9, where N is the number of ligands, $nlig$ is the number of atoms of each ligand and the function $interpolate$ performs the calculation of the electrostatic potential for each atom.

4.4.1.2 ES energy calculation on GPU

We describe in this part the different strategies studied for the GPU implementation. All designs have in common that one thread calculates the energy of only one atom. The threads are organized in blocks of fixed size $numThreads$, being this an important optimization parameter.

1. **GM** (use of device memory): In this initial design the whole grid is stored in the GPU device memory. No additional optimizations are implemented.
2. **ROI** (truncation to the grid around the ligand): In this strategy we have implemented some optimizations with respect to the previous version (GM). In order to reduce the CPU-GPU data transfer time, we can take advantage of the fact that we only need to access the grid positions in the volume where the ligand is enclosed. Thus, we can define a region of interest (ROI) of the grid around the ligand and send only that part to the GPU instead of the whole grid.

3. **ZIP** (compression of the grid): In addition, we can shorten the CPU-GPU grid transfer time with the compression of the positions of the ligand atoms. For that purpose, we discretize the volume that encloses the ligands in another cubic regular grid, where each ligand atom is specified only by its grid cell index. The advantage of this approach is that if we perform a fine grain division, each atom can be conveniently represented by just 3 short integers (instead of the three doubles required for position) and reduce memory usage to a quarter.
4. **SM** and **TM** (use of shared and texture memories): We can benefit from the use of shared and texture memory to improve memory access. In the shared memory approach (SM), threads of a block cooperate to copy ROI of the grid to the shared memory in order to obtain a lower memory access penalization. It must be noticed that accessing grid data on SM is coalesced in order to leverage memory bandwith. Regarding texture memory (TM) approach, we can store protein grid into the texture memory unit (TMI), so that just accessing different memory indexes gives us directly the interpolated (NVIDIA, 2010) energy value for each atom.

Algorithm 10 GPU pseudocode for the calculation of the electrostatic potential

Host (CPU)

```
CopyDataCPUtoGPU(GridROI)
clig = compress(lig)
CopyDataCPUtoGPU(clig)
nBlocks := N * nlig/numThreads
Kernel <<< nBlocks, numThreads >>> (GridROI, clig, energy)
CopyDataFromGPUtoCPU(energy)
```

Kernel 1: ROI-TM-ZIP

```
for all nBlocks do
    dlig = decompress(clig[myAtom])
    ilig = positionToROICoordinates(ROIinfo, dlig)
    energy[myAtom] = accessToTextureMemory(GridROI, ilig)
end for
```

Kernel 2: ROI-SM-ZIP

```
for all nBlocks do
    copyDataToSM(GridROI)
    dlig = decompress(clig[myAtom])
    ilig = positionToROICoordinates(GridROI, dlig)
    energy[myAtom] = interpolate(GridROI, dlig, ilig)
end for
```

Kernels shown in Algorithm 10 describe two different mixed groups of optimizations based on the previous strategies. In both Kernels, the host sends the ROI of the grid and the compressed ligand atom positions to the GPU. In Kernel 1 of Algorithm 10, each thread decompresses the coordinates of the corresponding atom and calculates its coordinates in the ROI coordinates system. Next, it performs interpolation in the TMI. In Kernel 2 of Algorithm 10, each thread also decompresses coordinates but the interpolation function is implemented in the code as described. Finally, energy values are copied back to CPU.

4.4.2 Grid spacing and interpolation accuracy

Figure 9 shows how grid spacing d influences accuracy in the different interpolation procedures. We wondered about the smallest possible value of d that yields good accuracy

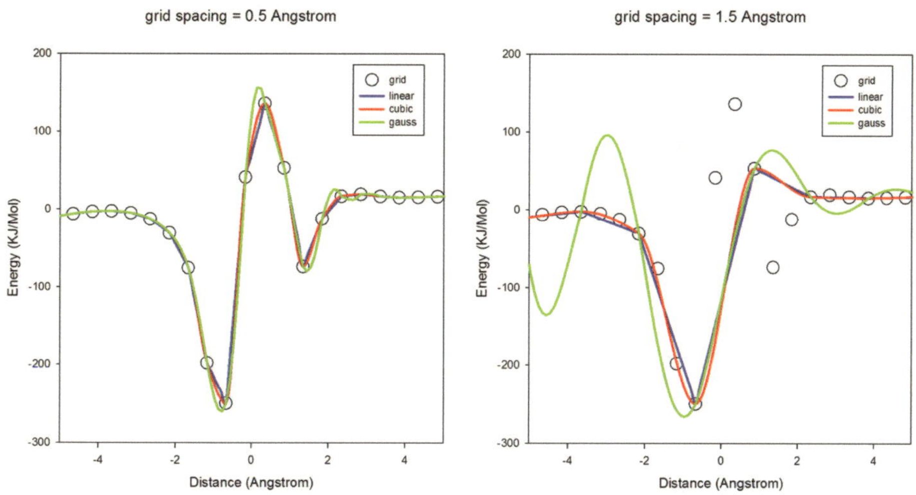

Fig. 9. Interpolation results obtained in a part of the grid streptavidin-biotin for grid spacing values of 0.5 (left picture) and 1.5 (right picture) Å, and using different interpolation procedures. For clarity of the comparison we show the values for the grid points pertaining to a grid with a spacing of 0.5 Å.

and that uses the less possible number of points for the grid, and therefore memory. We found that a value of $d = 0.5$ Å gives good accuracy for the three interpolation methods. Smaller values of d do not improve accuracy significantly while they require more memory (it depends on $(1/d)^3$). From the other side, higher values of d, like 1.5 Å yield unacceptable results for all studied interpolation methods in the rugged parts of the curve, which happens often due to the typical charge distribution in proteins. Therefore we accepted a value of $d = 0.5$ Å as optimal. Regarding the interpolation procedure we discarded the Gauss interpolation given its worst results in the rugged parts of the curve, if we compare it with cubic and linear interpolations, which yield similar accuracy. We finally decided to use only the latter given its lower computational cost. We also discarded interpolation methods of higher order since in the ROI strategy (grid is reduced around the ligand) they would not be able to access grid points out of ROI, yielding wrong results.

4.4.3 Analysis and performance of the sequential code

In Figure 10(B), we can see the timing results obtained for the sequential code in a ligand database screening with 2000 ligands. The trilinear interpolation needs to access eight adjacent cells of a ligand atom positions. It implies two memory accesses to four different rows of the grid. Furthermore, we cannot exploit the use of the cache due to the fact that the atoms are spread in random positions in the 3D space. Therefore most of the RAM accesses represent a bottleneck. Nevertheless, we have used this grid Kernel as starting point and investigated how to adapt it to the GPU architecture, since it is widely used in most biomolecular simulation methods. An additional reason is the 150 to 200 speedups in the sequential version versus the full kernel (Guerrero et al., 2011) for several grid densities and size ranges of rigid proteins. Besides, the GPU computational time is divided in Figure10(A) between time

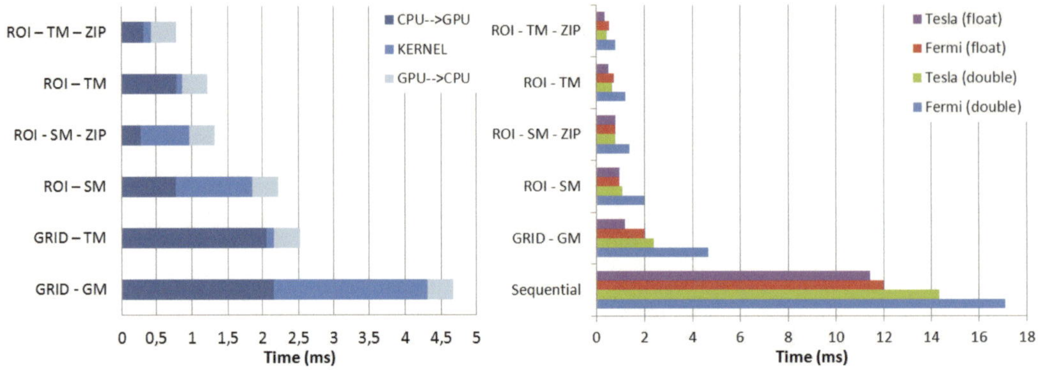

Fig. 10. (A) Comparison of running times for the sequential and GPU implementations. Protein studied is streptavidin and the screening was performed using a ligand database containing 2000 ligands, each one containing around 32 atoms. (B) Total running times for the two GPUs used in our study in float and double precision.

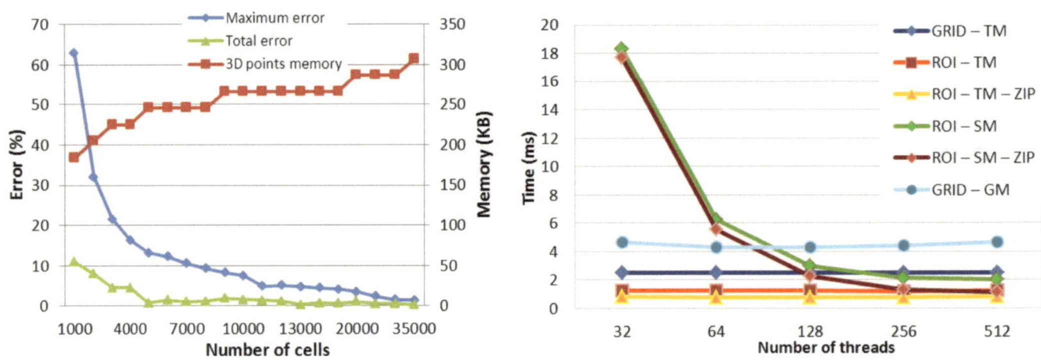

Fig. 11. (A) Values of the maximum and total error per atom obtained when using the compressed grid for representing the ligand database for several values of the number of cells and memory consumption in KB (B) Influence of the number of threads per block on the running time for the different implementation strategies studied.

dedicated to computation and memory transfers between CPU and GPU through PCI Express bus.

4.4.4 Compression of the ligand database atomic positions

In Figure 11(A) we can observe how the number of cells influences the error for the calculation of the electrostatic potential. As one would expect, increasing the number of cells reduces on average the maximum error for the calculation of the potential per atom, and the same for the total error. A maximum error of 0.25% is obtained when we use 35000 cells to compress the whole ligand database. At the same time, memory consumption increases only linearly given the efficiency of the compression method used and only around 300 KB are needed to store the whole ligand database.

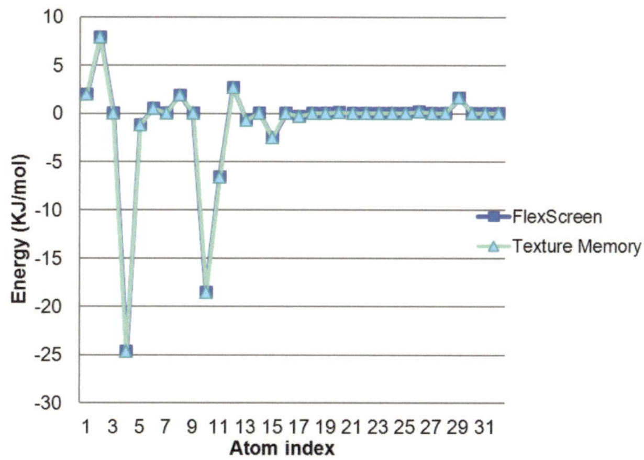

Fig. 12. Value of the electrostatic potential calculated for each atom of biotin in the binding pocket of streptavidin comparing the grid approach used in FlexScreen and using the Texture Memory of the GPU.

4.4.5 Threads per block

We have also investigated the influence of the number of threads per block as can be seen in Figure 11(B). Since the designs ROI-SM and ROI-SM-ZIP use the shared memory, they are more affected by the value of the block size than the others. If the number of threads per block is smaller than the ROI size, threads need to perform too many iterations to copy the whole ROI into the shared memory while the high bandwidth memory is unused. For a number of threads per block higher than the ROI size, the memory access bandwidth is improved because there are many simultaneous memory accesses. The global and texture memory are cached (only in the Fermi architecture) and the data copy is performed automatically in background independently of the number of threads. As a consecuence we have chosen a number of threads equal to 512 as optimal for the shared memory designs.

4.4.6 Texture memory

In the TM strategy we have first checked whether we obtain the same interpolation results than in the sequential version and this is confirmed in Figure 12. We can also see how the use of this memory unit decreases considerably the time needed for the calculation of the interpolation. It is clearly shown in Figure 10(A) in cases GRID-GM to GRID-TM and ROI-SM or ROI-SM-ZIP to ROI-TM. Therefore it is a good idea to use always the TMI when linear interpolation is required. Finally, if we look at Figure 10(A) it is clear that ROI-TM-ZIP and ROI-SM-ZIP offer the best performance since they combine all the best advantages from the previous strategies.

4.4.7 Floating point accuracy influence on different GPUs

We have also performed this study in several NVIDIA GPUs, both in simple and double precision, in order to check how the architectural design affects performance and precision. In Figure 10(B) we can observe that on average, Tesla GPU runs faster than Fermi GPU. For both cases the running times are smaller working on single than in double floating point precision, as one would expect. In the results obtained in the different GPU strategies presented, Tesla also outperforms Fermi due to the higher number of cores (448 versus 352). This is more accurate in the cases like GRID-GM where interpolation computations take a high percentage of the total running time.

4.5 MURCIA: Implicit solvation and molecular visualization

It is very important in clinical research to determine the safety and effectiveness of current drugs and to accelerate findings in basic research (discovery of new leads and active compounds) into meaningful health outcomes. Both objectives imply to be able to process the vast amount of protein structure data available in biological databases like PDB and also derived from genomic data using techniques as homology modelling (Sanchez & Sali, 1998). Screenings in lab and compound optimization are expensive and slow methods, but bioinformatics can vastly help clinical research for the mentioned purposes by providing prediction of the toxicity of drugs and activity in non-tested targets, by evolving discovered active compounds into drugs for the clinical trials. All this can be done thanks to the availability of bioinformatics tools and Virtual Screening (VS) methods that allow to test all required hypothesis before clinical trials. Nevertheless, VS methods fail to make good toxicity and activity predictions since they are constrained by the access to computational resources; even the nowadays fastest VS methods cannot process large biological databases in a reasonable time-frame. This imposes, thus a serious limitation in many areas of translational research.

We have previously studied how exploitation of last generation massively parallel hardware architectures like GPUs can tremendously overcome this problem accelerating the required calculations and allowing the introduction of improvements in the biophysical models not affordable in the past (Perez Sanchez & Wenzel, 2011). Between the most relevant computationally intensive kernels present in current VS methods, we may highlight the calculation of the molecular surface in terms of the solvent accessible surface area (SASA). We can model efficiently solvation in an implicit way by the calculation of SASA and posterior consideration of the hydrophobic and hydrophilic character of individual atoms (Eisenberg & McLachlan, 1986), being this method widely applied nowadays in protein structure prediction and protein-ligand binding. There have been several efforts to develop a fast method for the SASA calculation. To the best of our knowledge, the fastest method nowadays is POWERSASA (Klenin et al., 2011). Its running time depends linearly on the number of atoms of the molecule. We propose a new method called MURCIA (Molecular Unburied Rapid Calculation of Individual Areas) that uses the GPU as underlying hardware and which runs around 15 times faster than POWERSASA for the usual proteins that we found in most VS methods, with less than 25000 atoms. Another advantage of MURCIA is that it can rapidly provide molecular surface information useful for fast visualization in several molecular graphics programs.

4.5.1 SASA calculation using atomic grids

All atoms of the molecule are specified by their centers and SASA radii, which depend on their Van der Waals radius, and therefore on their atomic type, plus the water molecule radius. MURCIA calculates individual SASA values through the next three Kernels:

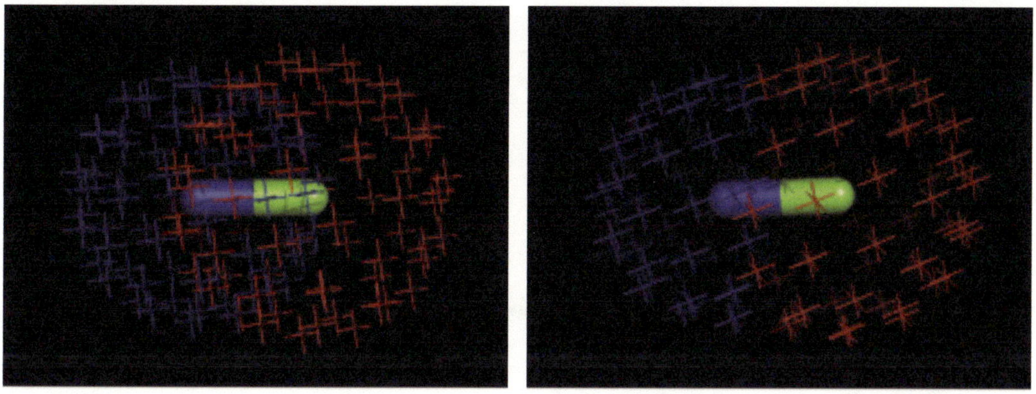

Fig. 13. Atomic grids for a molecule with two atoms (a) both grids overlap, situation previous to the SASA calculation, and (b) only non-buried grid points are shown

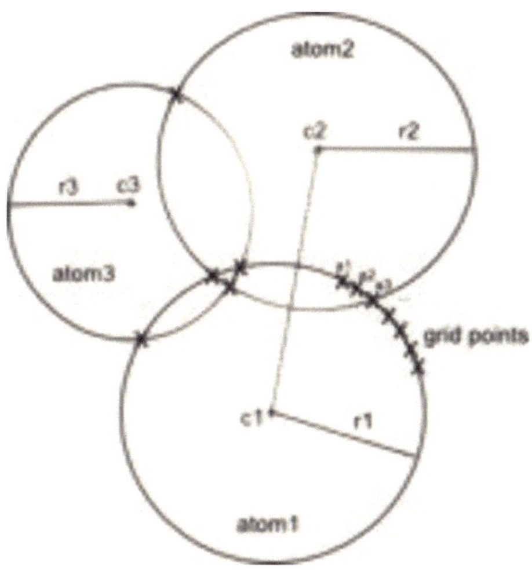

Fig. 14. Depiction in 2D of the SASA calculation in MURCIA

1. *GenGrid*: we build a grid of points around each atom following the procedure developed by Lebedev & Laikov (1999) for the numerical integration over a sphere. This grid guarantees a high precision in integrations, using a very low number of grid points over an unit sphere. In our case we use 72 points. An example of the grid is shown in Figure 13(a).
2. *Neighbours*: we calculate the list of its closest neighbours for each atom. The distance threshold is equal two times the highest value of the highest SASA radii. Atoms are sorted in the lists starting from the closest ones.
3. *Out points*: as depicted in Figure 14 for each atom i,, we perform the following calculation for each grid point k; we calculate squared distance to the first neighbour atom j of the list. If this distance is smaller than the SASA radius of atom j, then we flag this grid point as buried. Otherwise we continue the same procedure calculating distances versus the other atoms of the list. If the grid point k is not eventually flagged as buried, then it is stored as contributor to SASA for atom i. Once this procedure is finished for all grid points of

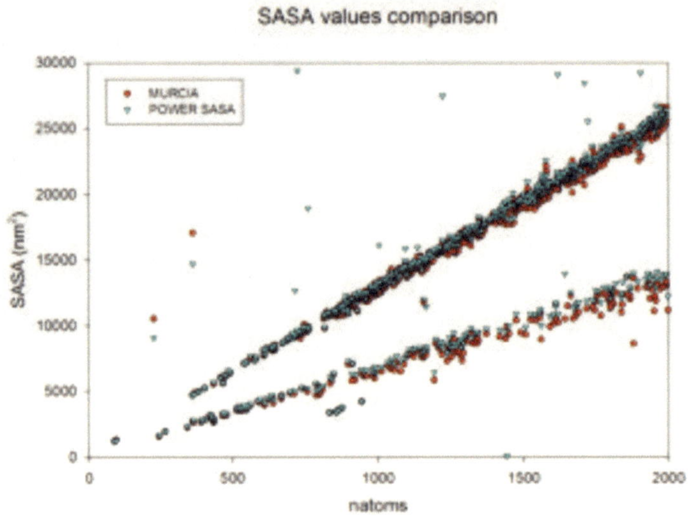

Fig. 15. Comparison of the SASA values calculated by POWERSASA and MURCIA. A diverse set of the PDB database was used for the calculations.

atom i, we will have n non-buried grid points, and individual SASA for this atom will be calculated according to a $(n/72)$ fraction of the sphere surface of radius corresponding to the SASA radius of this atom. At the same time, all coordinates of non-buried grid points are stored for posterior molecular visualization. The same procedure is applied to all atoms i of the molecule. An example of the resulting non-buried grid points is shown in Figure 13(b).

4.5.2 GPU implementation

We used the version 4.0 of the CUDA programming model (NVIDIA, 2011) in our parallel implementation with a NVIDIA Tesla C2050 GPU. In order to obtain speedup measurements versus the sequential counterpart version, an Intel Xeon E5450 cluster was used. This model allows writing parallel programs for GPUs using extensions of the C language. We describe here how the previous kernels are implemented on the GPU:

1. *GenGrid*: It generates atomic grids from the molecular input file. It divides the number of calculation for atoms into CUDA blocks, and assigns a number of threads per block proportional to the number of grid points per atom (72), so each thread computes only one grid point per atom.
2. *Neighbours*: It creates one CUDA block per atom and a variable number of threads per block. Each thread computes for each atom i the distances to the other atoms j. All threads from a block cooperate together to calculate all its neighbours using CUDA shared memory for storing variables commons to all threads of a block.
3. *Out Points*: It establishes the values of number of blocks and threads per block in the same way as the GenGrid kernel does. Each thread computes only distances between only one grid point and all of its neighbours.

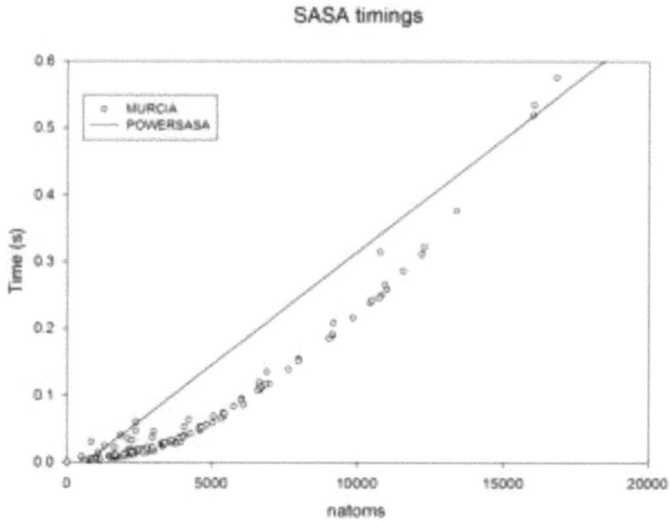

Fig. 16. Comparison of timings for SASA calculation using MURCIA and POWERSASA (since its dependence with the number of atoms is linear and for the sake of clarity, a solid line is used to represent its timings results). A diverse set of the PDB database was used for the calculations.

4.5.3 Performance evaluation

In order to check the accuracy of our method, we check MURCIA calculations with previous POWERSASA results (Klenin 2011). Figure 15 shows an overall good concordance between both methods. POWERSASA uses a very accurate method for the calculation of SASA. There are some cases where MURCIA deviates from the POWERSASA ones. We think this is due to the insufficient number of points (72) used for the atomic grids.

Figure 16 shows a performance comparison between MURCIA and POWERSASA. In the interval 10 to 17000 atoms, MURCIA runs faster than POWERSASA, achieving maximum speedups of 15x. For bigger molecules (20000-100000 atoms) POWERSASA runs faster than MURCIA. We have also checked that MURCIA runs around 30 times faster than MSMS (Sanner et al., 1996).

We have shown in this Section a fast and efficient method for the SASA calculation, implemented on GPU hardware, and which can also be used for fast visualization of molecular surfaces using information calculated for the non-buried atomic surfaces. Nevertheless, the method can be improved since more dense grids influences on the precision of the SASA calculation. Also, the main bottleneck of the program resides in the calculation of neighbours; a better strategy, which calculates much faster the neighbour's list might help considerably. Finally, MURCIA speedups visualization of molecular surfaces in some molecular graphics programs (VMD, Chimera, Pymol).

5. Conclusions and perspectives

After having shown current tendencies in these fields and also our main contributions, we think that the investigations on the improvement of the computational performance of

VS methods on GPUs will be also of high technological interest. Knowledge obtained in the works described here will be transferred to another scientists to port another scientific applications to the next generation of GPUs. So the results obtained in these research lines will offer major technological advantages: (i) performance offered by new parallel architectures will be unveiled; and (ii) cheap hardware equipment will be purchased instead of high-end expensive supercomputers. GPUs are likely to play a very important role in the next generation of VS methods. Thanks to the improvements obtained by implementation and optimization of VS methods in GPUs it will be possible to increase the details in simulations so that more refined and computationally expensive methods will be available at low cost. Supercomputing will be accessible for everyone, and scientific knowledge will advance faster. Techniques such as MD and QM methods, not widely used before due to their high computational cost, will become regular parts of VS methods. Global throughput of VS methods will increase and it will be possible to simulate more and longer trajectories within shorter times. It will be possible to use more accurate thermodynamic methods and compute free energies. Free-energy calculations will move away from individual predictions to form part of high-throughput VS methods.

6. References

Agullo, E., Demmel, J., Dongarra, J., Hadri, B., Kurzak, J., Langou, J., Ltaief, H., Luszczek, P. & Tomov, S. (2009). Numerical linear algebra on emerging architectures: The PLASMA and MAGMA projects, *Journal of Physics: Conference Series* 180(1): 012037. URL: *http://dx.doi.org/10.1088/1742-6596/180/1/012037*

Amdahl, G. M. (1967). Validity of the single processor approach to achieving large scale computing capabilities, *Proceedings of the April 18-20, 1967, spring joint computer conference*, AFIPS '67 (Spring), ACM, New York, NY, USA, pp. 483–485. URL: *http://doi.acm.org/10.1145/1465482.1465560*

ATI/AMD (2011). ATI Stream Webpage. `http://www.amd.com/US/PRODUCTS/TECHNOLOGIES/STREAM-TECHNOLOGY/Pages/st%ream-technology.aspx`.

Bohn, C.-A. (1998). Kohonen Feature Mapping through Graphics Hardware, *Proceedings of International Conference on Computational Intelligence and Neurosciences*, ICCIN 98, pp. 64–67.

Bursulaya, B. D., Totrov, M., Abagyan, R. & Brooks, C. L. (2003). Comparative study of several algorithms for flexible ligand docking., *J Comput Aided Mol Des* 17(11): 755–763. URL: *http://view.ncbi.nlm.nih.gov/pubmed/15072435*

Cecilia, J. M., García, J. M., Ujaldón, M., Nisbet, A. & Amos, M. (2011). Parallelization strategies for ant colony optimisation on gpus, *NIDISC '2011: 14th International Workshop on Nature Inspired Distributed Computing. Proc. 25th International Parallel and Distributed Processing Symposium (IPDPS 2011)*, Anchorage (Alaska), USA.

Cerutti, D. S., Duke, R. E., Darden, T. A. & Lybrand, T. P. (2009). Staggered Mesh Ewald: An Extension of the Smooth Particle-Mesh Ewald Method Adding Great Versatility, *Journal Of Chemical Theory And Computation* 5(9): 2322–2338.

CUD (2011). The CUDA Zone website. `http://www.nvidia.com/object/cuda_home_new.html`.

Dorigo, M. (1992). *Optimization, Learning and Natural Algorithms*, PhD thesis, Politecnico di Milano, Italy.

Eisenberg, D. & McLachlan, A. D. (1986). Solvation energy in protein folding and binding., *Nature* 319(6050): 199–203.

England, J. N. (1978). A System for Interactive Modeling of Physical Curved Surface Objects, *Proceedings of the 5th annual Conference on Computer Graphics and Interactive Techniques*, SIGGRAPH 78, ACM, pp. 336–340.

Feng, Z.-w., Tian, X.-h. & Chang, S. (2010). A Parallel Molecular Docking Approach Based on Graphic Processing Unit, *Bioinformatics and Biomedical Engineering (iCBBE), 2010 4th International Conference on*, pp. 1–4.

Fischer, B., Basili, S., Merlitz, H. & Wenzel, W. (2007). Accuracy of binding mode prediction with a cascadic stochastic tunneling method, *Proteins: Structure, Function, and Bioinformatics* 68(1): 195–204.

Friesner, R. A. & Banks, J. L. (2004). Glide: A New Approach for Rapid, Accurate Docking and Scoring. 1. Method and Assessment of Docking Accuracy, *Journal of Medicinal Chemistry* 47(7): 1739–1749.
URL: *http://dx.doi.org/10.1021/jm0306430*

Garland, M. & Kirk, D. B. (2010). Understanding throughput-oriented architectures, *Commun. ACM* 53: 58–66.

Garland, M., Le Grand, S., Nickolls, J., Anderson, J., Hardwick, J., Morton, S., Phillips, E., Zhang, Y. & Volkov, V. (2008). Parallel computing experiences with cuda, *IEEE Micro* 28: 13–27.

Graham, S. L., Kessler, P. B. & McKusick, M. K. (2004). gprof: a call graph execution profiler, *SIGPLAN Not.* 39: 49–57.
URL: *http://doi.acm.org/10.1145/989393.989401*

Guerrero, G., Pérez-Sánchez, H., Wenzel, W., Cecilia, J. M. & García, J. M. (2011). Effective parallelization of non-bonded interactions kernel for virtual screening on gpus, *5th International Conference on Practical Applications of Computational Biology; Bioinformatics (PACBB 2011)*, Vol. 93, Springer Berlin / Heidelberg, pp. 63–69.

Harris, M. J. (2002). Analysis of Error in a CML Diffusion Operation, *Technical Report TR02-015*, University of North Carolina.

Harvey, M. J. & De Fabritiis, G. (2009). An Implementation of the Smooth Particle Mesh Ewald Method on GPU Hardware, *Journal of Chemical Theory and Computation* 5(9): 2371–2377.
URL: *http://dx.doi.org/10.1021/ct900275y*

Hetényi, C. & van der Spoel, D. (2002). Efficient docking of peptides to proteins without prior knowledge of the binding site., *Protein science : a publication of the Protein Society.* 11(7): 1729–1737.
URL: *http://dx.doi.org/10.1110/ps.0202302*

Hoff, III, K. E., Zaferakis, A., Lin, M. & Manocha, D. (2001). Fast and simple 2D geometric proximity queries using Graphics hardware, *Proceedings of the 2001 Symposium on Interactive 3D Graphics*, I3D 01, ACM, pp. 145–148.

Hopf, M. & Ertl, T. (1999). Accelerating 3D convolution using Graphics hardware (case study), *Proceedings of the Conference on Visualization*, VIS 99, IEEE Computer Society Press, pp. 471–474.

Hopf, M. & Thomas, T. (1999). Hardware Based Wavelet Transformations, *Proceedings of Workshop on Vision, Modeling, and Visualization*, pp. 317–328.

Hui-fang, L., Qing, S., Jian, Z. & Wei, F. (2010). Evaluation of various inverse docking schemes in multiple targets identification., *Journal of molecular graphics & modelling* 29(3): 326–330.

Hwu, W.-m. W. (ed.) (2011). *GPU Computing Gems: Emerald Edition*, Morgan Kaufmann.

Jorgensen, W.L., M. D. T.-R. J. (1996). Development and testing of the opls all-atom force field on conformational energetics and properties of organic liquids, *Journal of the American Chemical Society* 118(45): 11225–11236.

Kannan, S. & Ganji, R. (2010). Porting Autodock to CUDA, *Evolutionary Computation (CEC), 2010 IEEE Congress on* pp. 1–8.

Kedem, G. & Ishihara, Y. (1999). Brute force attack on UNIX passwords with SIMD Computer, *Proceedings of the 8th Conference on USENIX Security Symposium*, USENIX Association, pp. 8–8.

Kirk, D. B. & Hwu, W.-m. W. (2010). *Programming Massively Parallel Processors: A Hands-on Approach*, Morgan Kaufmann.

Klenin, K. V., Tristram, F., Strunk, T. & Wenzel, W. (2011). Derivatives of molecular surface area and volume: Simple and exact analytical formulas., *Journal of Computational Chemistry* 32(12): 2647–2653.

Klöckner, A., Pinto, N., Lee, Y., Catanzaro, B., Ivanov, P. & Fasih, A. (2011). PyCUDA and PyOpenCL: A Scripting-Based Approach to GPU Run-Time Code Generation, *ArXiv e-prints* .
URL: *http://arxiv.org/abs/0911.3456*

Kokh, D. B., Wade, R. C. & Wenzel, W. (2011). Receptor flexibility in small-molecule docking calculations, *Wiley Interdisciplinary Reviews: Computational Molecular Science* 1(2): 298–314.
URL: *http://dx.doi.org/10.1002/wcms.29*

Kokh, D. B. & Wenzel, W. (2008). Flexible side chain models improve enrichment rates in in silico screening, *Journal of Medicinal Chemistry* 51(19): 5919–5931.

Korb, O., Stützle, T. & Exner, T. (2006). PLANTS: Application of Ant Colony Optimization to Structure-Based Drug Design, *in* M. Dorigo, L. Gambardella, M. Birattari, A. Martinoli, R. Poli & T. Stützle (eds), *Ant Colony Optimization and Swarm Intelligence*, Vol. 4150 of *Lecture Notes in Computer Science*, Springer Berlin / Heidelberg, Berlin, Heidelberg, chapter 22, pp. 247–258.

Korb, O., Stützle, T. & Exner, T. E. (2011). Accelerating molecular docking calculations using graphics processing units., *Journal of chemical information and modeling* 51(4): 865–876.

Larsen, E. S. & McAllister, D. (2001). Fast matrix multiplies using Graphics hardware, *Proceedings of the 2001 ACM/IEEE Conference on Supercomputing*, Supercomputing 01, ACM, pp. 55–55.

Lebedev, V. I. & Laikov, D. N. (1999). A quadrature formula for the sphere of the 131st algebraic order of accuracy, *Doklady Mathematics* 59(3): 477–481.

Lengyel, J., Reichert, M., Donald, B. R. & Greenberg, D. P. (1990). Real-time robot motion planning using rasterizing computer graphics hardware, *Proceedings of the 17th annual Conference on Computer Graphics and Interactive Techniques*, SIGGRAPH 90, ACM, pp. 327–335.

Lindholm, E., Kilgard, M. J. & Moreton, H. (2001). A user-programmable vertex engine, *Proceedings of the 28th annual Conference on Computer Graphics and Interactive Techniques*, SIGGRAPH 01, ACM, pp. 149–158.

Luebke, D. (2007). The Democratization of Parallel Computing. Keynote at International Conference on Supercomputing.

Luebke, D., Harris, M., Govindaraju, N., Lefohn, A., Houston, M., Owens, J., Segal, M., Papakipos, M. & Buck, I. (2006). GPGPU: General-Purpose Computation on Graphics hardware, *Proceedings of the 2006 ACM/IEEE Conference on Supercomputing*, SC 2006, ACM.

Manfrin, M., Birattari, M., Stützle, T. & Dorigo, M. (2006). Parallel ant colony optimization for the traveling salesman problem, *in* M. Dorigo, L. M. Gambardella, M. Birattari, A. Martinoli, R. Poli & T. Stützle (eds), *Ant Colony Optimization and Swarm Intelligence, 5th International Workshop, ANTS˜2006*, Vol. 4150 of *LNCS*, Springer Verlag, Berlin, Germany, pp. 224–234.

Meliciani, I., Perez Sanchez, H. & Wenzel, W. (2009). Analysis of the complex antithrombin/thrombin and alanine mutation of the complex antithrombin/heparin using two different docking approaches (poem, flexscreen).

Meng, E., Shoichet, B. & Kuntz, I. (1992). Automated Docking with Grid-Based Energy Evaluation, *Journal of Computational Chemistry* 13(4): 505–524.

Merlitz, H., Burghardt, B. & Wenzel, W. (2003). Application of the stochastic tunneling method to high throughput database screening, *Chemical physics letters* 370(1-2): 68–73.

Merlitz, H., Herges, T. & Wenzel, W. (2004). Fluctuation analysis and accuracy of a large-scalein silico screen, *Journal of Computational Chemistry* 25(13): 1568–1575.

Navarro-Fernandez, J., Martinez-Martinez, I., Perez-Sanchez, H., Meliciani, I., Wenzel, W., de la Morena-Barrio, M., Vicente, V. & Corral, J. (2010). Identification of a compound with enhanced capacity in the activation of antithrombin in presence of heparin.

Nguyen, H. (2007). *GPU Gems 3*, Addison-Wesley Professional.

NVIDIA (2009). *Whitepaper NVIDIA's Next Generation CUDA Compute Architecture: Fermi.*

NVIDIA (2010). *NVIDIA CUDA Programming Guide 4.0.*

NVIDIA (2011). *NVIDIA CUDA C Programming Guide 4.0.*

Owens, John, D., Luebke, David, Govindaraju, Naga, Harris, Mark, Kruger, Jens, Lefohn, Aaron, E., Purcell & Timothy, J. (2007). A Survey of General-Purpose Computation on Graphics Hardware, *Computer Graphics Forum* 26(1): 80–113.

Pérez-Sánchez, H. (2009). Implementation of an Effective Non-Bonded Interactions Kernel for Biomolecular Simulations on the Cell Processor, *Gesselschaft für Informatik* .

Perez Sanchez, H. & Wenzel, W. (2011). Optimization methods for virtual screening on novel computational architectures., *Current computer-aided drug design* 7(1): 44–52.

Pharr, M. & Fernando, R. (2005). *GPU Gems 2: Programming Techniques for High-Performance Graphics and General-Purpose Computation*, Addison-Wesley Professional.

Potmesil, M. & Hoffert, E. M. (1989). The Pixel Machine: A Parallel Image Computer, *Proceedings of the 16th annual Conference on Computer Graphics and Interactive Techniques*, SIGGRAPH 89, ACM, pp. 69–78.

Press, W. H., Teukolsky, S. A., Vetterling, W. T. & Flannery, B. P. (1992). *Numerical Recipes in C: The Art of Scientific Computing*, 2nd edn, Cambridge University Press, New York, NY, USA.

Rhoades, J., Turk, G., Bell, A., State, A., Neumann, U. & Varshney, A. (1992). Real-time procedural textures, *Proceedings of the 1992 Symposium on Interactive 3D Graphics*, I3D 92, ACM, pp. 95–100.

Roh, Y., Lee, J., Park, S. & Kim, J.-I. (2009). A molecular docking system using CUDA, *ICHIT '09: Proceedings of the 2009 International Conference on Hybrid Information Technology* .

Sanchez, R. & Sali, A. (1998). Large-Scale Protein Structure Modeling of the Saccharomyces cerevisiae Genome, *Proceedings Of The National Academy Of Sciences Of The United States Of America* 95(23): 13597–13602.

Sanders, J. & Kandrot, E. (2010). *CUDA by Example: An Introduction to General-Purpose GPU Programming*, Addison-Wesley Professional.

Sanner, M. F., Olson, A. J. & Spehner, J. C. (1996). Reduced surface: an efficient way to compute molecular surfaces., *Biopolymers* 38(3): 305–320.

Schneider, G. & Böhm, H. J. (2002). Virtual screening and fast automated docking methods., *Drug Discov Today* 7(1): 64–70.
URL: *http://view.ncbi.nlm.nih.gov/pubmed/11790605*

Stone, J. E., Phillips, J. C., Freddolino, P. L., Hardy, D. J., Trabuco, L. G. & Schulten, K. (2007). Accelerating molecular modeling applications with graphics processors, *Journal of Computational Chemistry* 28(16): 2618–2640.

Strzodka, R. (2002). Virtual 16 Bit Precise Operations an RGBA8 Textures, *Proceedings of the Vision, Modeling, and Visualization Conference*, VMV 2002, pp. 171–178.

Strzodka, R. (2004). *Hardware Efficient PDE Solvers in Quantized Image Processing*, PhD thesis, University of Duisburg-Essen.

Sukhwani, B. & Herbordt, M. (2010). Fast binding site mapping using GPUs and CUDA, *Parallel & Distributed Processing, Workshops and Phd Forum (IPDPSW), 2010 IEEE International Symposium on* pp. 1–8.

Thompson, C. J., Hahn, S. & Oskin, M. (2002). Using modern graphics architectures for general-purpose computing: a framework and analysis, *Proceedings of the 35th annual ACM/IEEE International Symposium on Microarchitecture*, MICRO 35, IEEE Computer Society Press, pp. 306–317.

Trendall, C. & Stewart, A. J. (2000). General calculations using graphics hardware with applications to interactive caustics, *Proceedings of the Eurographics Workshop on Rendering Techniques 2000*, Springer-Verlag, pp. 287–298.

Volkov, V. & Demmel, J. W. (2008). Benchmarking gpus to tune dense linear algebra, *Proceedings of the 2008 ACM/IEEE conference on Supercomputing*, SC '08, IEEE Press, Piscataway, NJ, USA, pp. 31:1–31:11.
URL: *http://portal.acm.org/citation.cfm?id=1413370.1413402*

Volkov, V. & Kazian, B. (2008). Fitting fft onto the g80 architecture, *Methodology* p. 6.

Wang, J., Deng, Y. & Roux, B. (2006). Absolute Binding Free Energy Calculations Using Molecular Dynamics Simulations with Restraining Potentials, *Biophys. J.* 91(8): 2798–2814.
URL: *http://dx.doi.org/10.1529/biophysj.106.084301*

Xing, L., Hodgkin, E., Liu, Q. & Sedlock, D. (2004). Evaluation and application of multiple scoring functions for a virtual screening experiment, *Journal of Computer-Aided Molecular Design* 18(5): 333–344.

Yang, H., Zhou, Q., Li, B., Wang, Y., Luan, Z., Qian, D. & Li, H. (2010). GPU Acceleration of Dock6's Amber Scoring Computation, *Advances in Computational Biology* 680: 497–511.

Yuriev, E., Agostino, M. & Ramsland, P. A. (2011). Challenges and advances in computational docking: 2009 in review, *Journal Of Molecular Recognition* 24(2): 149–164.

Zhang, C., Liu, S., Zhu, Q. & Zhou, Y. (2005). A knowledge-based energy function for protein-ligand, protein-protein, and protein-DNA complexes., *Journal of Medicinal Chemistry* 48(7): 2325–2335.

Part 3

Application Examples on Modeling Methods Implemented in Virtual Screening

3

CoMFA/CoMSIA and Pharmacophore Modelling as a Powerful Tools for Efficient Virtual Screening: Application to Anti-Leishmanial Betulin Derivatives

Leo Ghemtio, Yuezhou Zhang and Henri Xhaard
Centre for Drug Research, Faculty of Pharmacy, University of Helsinki, Finland

1. Introduction

Improvement of efficiency as well as speed and accuracy in the step of identification of chemicals that excerpt *in vitro* or *in vivo* activity would help reduce the huge investments made by pharmaceutical companies in drug development projects. Traditionally, *in silico* high-throughput screening techniques, either based on protein binding site fitting (docking) or ligand similarity, are used to select the most promising molecules from large chemical libraries.(Ling & Xuefeng, 2008; Stahura & Bajorath, 2004; Tuccinardi, 2009; Villoutreix et al., 2009) Nonetheless, these computational techniques are hampered by high rates of false positives and high demand in computational resources.(Ghemtio et al., 2010) To avoid these shortcomings, predictive three-dimensional (3D) quantitative structure–activity relationship (3D-QSAR) combined with pharmacophore computational models coupled to ligand-based three-dimensional virtual screening (3D-VS) are becoming increasingly popular.(Clark, 2009; Ekins et al., 2007; Ghemtio et al., 2010; Kirchmair et al., 2008; Kirchmair et al., 2008; Langer & Hoffmann, 2001; Lengauer, 2004; Rognan, 2010; Sippl, 2002; Spitzer et al., 2010; Tropsha & Golbraikh, 2007). For example, previously, combination of 3D-QSAR studies and 3D-VS have been successfully applied for screening large collection of natural products and synthetic chemicals.(Clark, 2009; Liu et al., Nagarajan et al., 2010; Sippl, 2002; Spitzer et al., 2010)

The general idea is that after building a 3D-QSAR model that predicts usually the binding constant or *in vitro* biological activities of compounds from their 3D chemical properties, the 3D pharmacophoric representation of the shared chemical features that are most important towards activity can be used as a constraint for 3D-VS. Generally, a binding constant is accurately measured experimentally, relates to a single type of molecular event, and therefore is a suitable source of data for 3D-QSAR modeling. There is however a large gap between the binding constant to given protein and any therapeutic effect that may be provided by a compound. *In vitro* activities relate in many cases to a compound binding to several target proteins or to other cellular effects but can still be useful for 3D-QSAR. *In vivo* activities on the other hand are the sum of so many complex and mechanistically different processes that they are not a reasonable source of data for 3D-QSAR modeling.

Here, we aim to interpret the *in vitro* anti-leishmanial activities of a set of 24 betulin derivatives (BDIs), i.e. compounds derived from a betulin scaffold, as well as to screen for novel potentially interesting chemicals. Leishmaniases are diseases caused by protozoan parasites that affect millions of people in more than 88 countries worldwide.(Alakurtti et al., 2010) Several drugs are available for the treatment of these diseases, for example pentavalent antimony compounds derived from the heavy metal antimony (Sb), pentamidine or amphotericin B, and miltefosine compounds. However, these drugs present severe side effects, parasite resistance, are too expensive for use in less-developed countries, and for some are dangerous to use in pregnant women.(Pink et al., 2005) There is therefore an urgent need for the development of safe chemicals for the treatment of all clinical forms of leishmaniasis. For this purpose, betulin derivatives are one of the most investigated classes of compounds. While the molecular mechanism of the inhibitory action of betulin derivatives on *Leishmania donovani* growth is to date unknown, several protein targets have been suggested including the Topoisomerase 2 enzyme. Betulins present several advantages that make them a very suitable class of compounds to run quantitative structure–activity relationship (SAR) studies and, despite their large size and hydrophobicity, to be investigated as a therapeutic class of compounds: a five-ring chemical scaffold allows a straightforward three dimensional superimposition, while the parent molecule can be extracted easily and in large quantities from the bark of birch tree, and is easily chemically modifiable at three sites. In addition to anti-Leishmania activity, betulin derivatives have shown anti-inflammatory, antimalarial and especially cytotoxic activity against several tumor cell lines by inducing apoptosis in cells.(Alakurtti et al., 2010; Alakurtti et al., 2006) Structure–activity relationship studies and pharmacological properties of betulin and its derivatives have been reviewed recently.(Alakurtti et al., 2006)

In this chapter, we have developed predictive 3D-QSAR models that help to interpret the *in vitro* anti-leishmanial activities of a small but consistent set of 24 betulin derivatives (the chemical structures are shown in Table 1). (Alakurtti et al., 2010). We first use two popular and well-studied 3D-QSAR methods; comparative molecular field analysis (CoMFA)(Cramer et al., 1988), and comparative molecular similarity indices analysis (CoMSIA)(Klebe et al., 1994) implemented in Sybyl-X to construct predictive 3D-QSAR models that predict the activities of betulin derivatives from a small but consistent dataset. In these methods the proper alignment of molecular structures across the series and the selection of the bioactive conformation are critical yet often problematic. The 3D-QSAR models developed here should serve as a useful tool to predict the inhibitory properties of untested compounds and therefore help to guide synthesis for the further development of more potent anti-leishmanial inhibitors. Secondly, the 3D-QSAR models together with compound 3D structures were used to develop 3D pharmacophore models that describe the chemical features most important for activity, using the GALAHAD (Genetic Algorithm with Linear Assignment of Hypermolecular Alignment of Database)(Richmond et al., 2006) implemented in Sybyl-X. Only the five most active molecules well predicted by the 3D-QSAR models were used for pharmacophore development. Thirdly, these pharmacophore models were used as 3D constraints to query two libraries for new chemical structures, one containing 120.000 compounds and the other containing 240.000 compounds.

2. Materials and methods

2.1 Compounds and biological data

The molecular structures and biological data used in this study were retrieved from a series of 24 betulin derivatives developed by Alakurtti et al. The chemical structures and experimental activities are shown in Table 1.(Alakurtti et al., 2010) The biological activities are reported as the percent inhibition of *Leishmania donovani* axenic amastigotes growth at 50 μM of betulin derivatives and were used as dependent variables in this study. These represent the percentage of growth reduction of *Leishmania donovani* axenic amastigotes associated with adding 50 μM of betulin derivatives to the cells.

Other type of data, such as growth rate constants, would have been perhaps been more reliable for 3D-QSAR modeling but were not accessible to us at time of this study.

All pharmacological data were obtained from the same laboratory, eliminating the potential noise that might have been introduced by the pooling of data sets from different sources. The inhibition (I_{50}) percentage values were converted in negative logarithmic units (pI_{50}, M) using Sybyl-X. The CoMFA/CoMSIA models were developed using 16 compounds as training set, and externally validated using 8 compounds as test set (see Table 1). The compound set was randomly divided into a training set and a test set (distributed using a 2/3 and 1/3 rule). After this division, we checked that both sets represent equally well the chemical and biological properties of the whole data set. The range of pI_{50} values for both the training and test set spans at least three orders of magnitude (2.30-5.91), and in addition the biological activity values are well distributed over the entire range. The compound 18 is later used as a reference, since it is the most active.

Accounting for outliers, either activity outliers, i.e. similar compounds for which different activities have been recorded, or leverage outliers, i.e. compounds chemically dissimilar from the rest of the set, is an important step in any type of QSAR modelling. One of the main deficiencies of some chemical datasets is that they do not satisfy the hypothesis that similar compounds share similar biological activities or properties. Outliers may originate from genuine effects, i.e. activity cliffs, may be due to artifacts and errors in structure representation, may result from a poor identification of chemical similarity, or may come from a poor annotation of biological activity. In addition, outliers may originate from different molecular mechanisms of action that may involve seemingly similar compounds. Outlier detection and removal before proceeding to model development is the best way to avoid model instability with significant differences in external predictive power of models. (Tropsha, 2010).

In this study, the compounds in the dataset are based on the same betulin chemical scaffold and therefore should be chemically similar one to another. As we will show below, there is a chemical reason to suspect that a few compounds can use a mechanism of action based on formation of covalent adducts, a mechanism that is quite different from the other molecules in the set. Removing these outliers from training and test set clearly led to improved models. Interestingly enough, we first noticed these compounds being outliers based on CoMFA/CoMSIA modeling and only afterwards identified a reasonable molecular explanation for this behaviour.

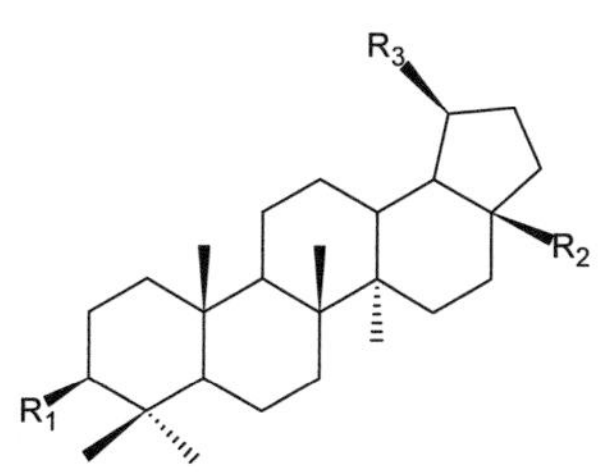

Compound	R1	R2	R3	pI_{50exp}	Prediction CoMFA pI_{50pred}	Prediction CoMSIA pI_{50pred}
			Training set			
1*	OH	CH2OH	CH3-C=CH2	4.03	4.11	3.94
2*	OH	CO2H	CH3-C=CH2	4.12	4.03	4.11
4*	**OH**	**CHO**	**CH3-C=CH2**	**4.55**	**4.60**	**4.49**
6	OH	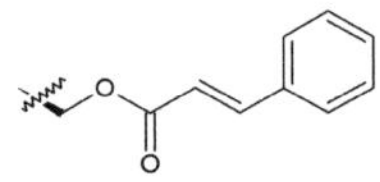	CH3-C=CH2	2.30	-	-
9	OH	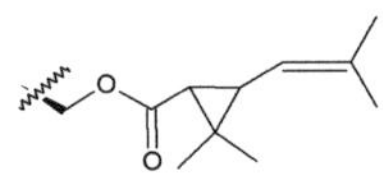	CH3-C=CH2	3.49	3.44	3.49
10	OH	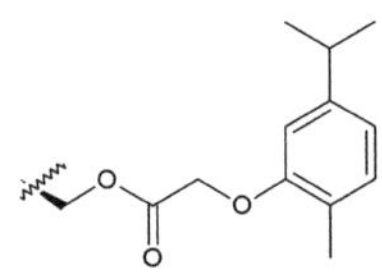	CH3-C=CH2	3.60	3.69	3.60
12	OH	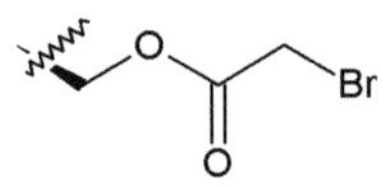	CH3-C=CH2	5.08	-	-
14	OAc	CH2OAc	CH3-C=CH2	2.30	2.30	2.20
15	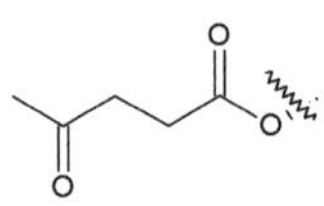	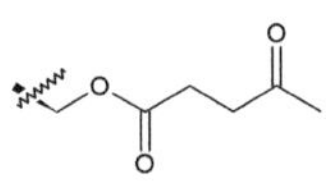	CH3-C=CH2	2.30	2.19	2.42
17*	O=	CHO	CH3-C=CH2	4.23	4.72	4.16
18*	**O=**	**CO2H**	**CH3-C=CH2**	**5.91**	**4.72**	**5.79**
20*	O=	CO2Me	CH3-C=CH2	4.12	4.67	4.28
21	**O=**	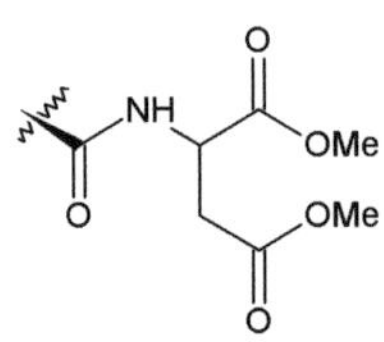	**CH3-C=CH2**	**4.65**	**4.81**	**4.67**
23*	-	CH2OH	CH3-C=CH2	3.48	3.82	3.41
24*	**OH**	**CH=NOH**	**CH3-C=CH2**	**4.65**	**4.59**	**4.77**
25*	**=NOH**	**CH=NOH**	**CH3-C=CH2**	**4.73**	**4.44**	**4.80**
			Testing set			
7	OH	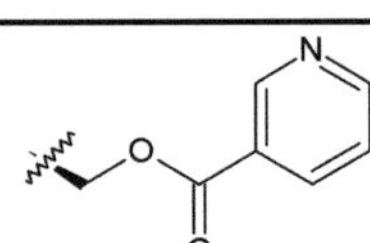	CH3-C=CH2	3.28	3.91	3.75

8	OH	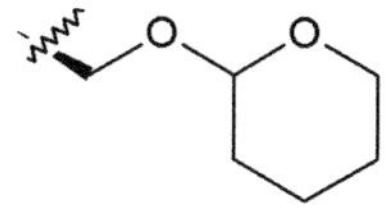	CH3-C=CH2	3.37	3.62	3.83
11	OH	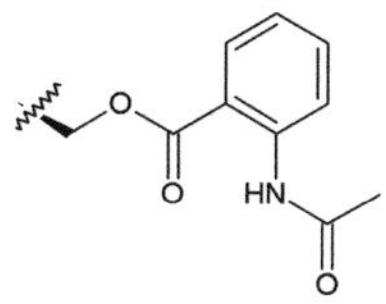	CH3-C=CH2	4.46	4.63	4.04
13*	OAc	OH	CH3-C=CH2	4.07	4.05	3.95
16*	O=	CH2OAc	CH3-C=CH2	4.13	4.28	3.85
19*	O=	CO2H	CH3CHCH2	4.71	4.34	5.01
22	O=	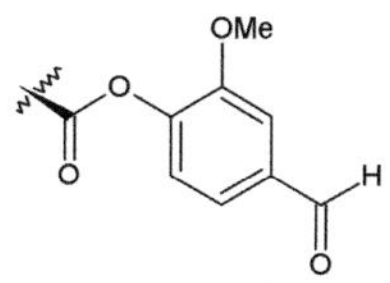	CH3-C=CH2	2.30	2.64	2.34
26*	OAc	CN	CH3-C=CH2	4.52	4.18	4.05

Table 1. Experimental and predicted Leishmanial growth inhibitory activities of Betulin derivatives used in the study. The first group is the training set and the second group is the test set. Compounds used for pharmacophore modelling are shown in bold. When the set was used as control (see section 3.3) in pharmacophore based virtual screening 3D search, the compounds marked with (*) were retrieved.

2.2 Generating the molecular structures and conformational analysis

The molecular structures of betulin derivatives were sketched using Sybyl-X v1.2 software(Tripos International, St. Louis). The fragment libraries in Sybyl-X database were used as building blocks to build three-dimensional structures of functional groups added to the betulin scaffold. A single conformation for each chemical was randomly picked, but it should be noted that conformational space is available for the R groups while the betulin scaffold is rigid. All the structures were assigned Gasteiger-Huckel charges and energy minimized using the standard Tripos force field (Powell method and 0.05 kcal/(mol.Å) energy gradient convergence criteria) (Tripos International, St. Louis). These conformations were used as starting conformations to perform the following 3D-QSAR and pharmacophore studies.

2.3 3D-QSAR models

3D-QSAR methodologies such as CoMFA/CoMSIA, aim to correlate biological activities with the three dimensional structures of compounds. Among these, comparative molecular field analysis (CoMFA) is widely used and historically the first, and has been improved since. CoMFA is restricted to electrostatic fields and therefore accounts only for the enthalpic contribution of binding(Klebe et al., 1994), with the underlying idea that if the aligned molecules share global shape and location in the 3D lattice, the entropic contributions to the free energy of binding to a molecular target are expected to be similar.(Perkins et al., 2003) The CoMFA Lennard-Jones and Coulomb potentials are sharp and may introduce errors in scaling, alignment sensitivity, and interpretation of contours. (Bostrom et al., 2003) In order to improve these shortcomings, the comparative molecular similarity indices (CoMSIA) methods have been developed that make usage in addition to the electrostatic fields of hydrophobic fields, supposed to account better for differences in the entropic contribution to binding free energy, hydrogen bonding fields, as well as use smoother potentials based on Gaussian functions, which are less sensible to variation in alignment and lead to more interpretable contours.(Buolamwini & Assefa, 2003)

CoMFA/CoMSIA alignment rules

The three-dimensional alignment of chemical structures is one of the most important steps in 3D-QSAR methodologies. For a set of congeneric chemicals, an optimal alignment of a set of molecules can be defined as the alignment that achieves the maximum superposition of steric and electrostatic fields. In CoMFA/CoMSIA modeling, significant and relevant results should be expected only for valid alignments. There are multiple strategies available in the literature depending on the specificity of each dataset for compound alignment as well as resources. Commonly used among commercial solutions are Sybyl-X 1.2 database alignment, Sybyl-X 1.2 atom fit alignment, SYBYL-X 1.2 Surflex-Sim(Jain, 2004), BRUTUS(Rönkkö et al., 2006; Tervo et al., 2005), or for freely available softwares ShaEP(Vainio et al., 2009). These tools can be used separately or together to identify the effect of the alignment on the final prediction. In reality, the alignment that we aim to recreate should reflect the superimposition that the set of compounds adopt when binding to a given molecular target; however a given set of molecules may bind in different ways when confronted to another binding site. In the present study, no binding site is available to guide the molecular alignment of betulin derivatives. We can however take advantage from the fact that the compounds used in our study are very similar and share a common five-member ring scaffold while they vary with the attached functional groups.

In this study, the alignment of training set was made with database alignment algorithms (Sybyl-X 1.2 database alignment) by using template compound (compound 18) as the basis for the alignment. Database alignment corresponds to the superposition of the common substructure shared by all molecules (Fig. 1). For superposition, compound 18 with the highest pI_{50} (5.91) was used as template molecule. All the five rings of the betulin scaffold were selected for superimposition and a rigid body superposition performed. The substituent R_3 is highly conformational flexible, however we did not select the individual conformations that would lead to an optimal superimposition of R_3. Optimizing this region would have required further work but could have lead to more predictive models.

CoMFA/CoMSIA fields calculation

The aligned training sets of molecules were positioned inside grid boxes with grid spacing value of 2 Å (default distance) in all Cartesian directions and CoMFA fields were calculated using the QSAR module of Sybyl-X(Tripos International, St. Louis). The interaction energies for each molecule were calculated at each grid point using probe atom: an sp^3 hybridized carbon atom with a van der Waals (vdW) radius of 1 Å and a +1 charge (default probe). The steric (vdW interaction) and electrostatic (Coulombic values) fields were calculated at each intersection on the regularly spaced grid. The cutoff value for both steric and electrostatic interaction was set to 30 kcal/mol. CoMSIA similarity index descriptors was derived using the same lattice boxes as those used in CoMFA calculations. Five physicochemical properties steric, electrostatic, hydrophobic, hydrogen bond donor and acceptor were evaluated using a common probe atom of 1 Å radius. In CoMSIA, the steric indices are related to the third power of the atomic radii, the electrostatic descriptors are derived from atomic partial charges, the hydrophobic fields are derived from atom-based parameters developed by Viswanadhan and co-workers(Viswanadhan et al., 1989), and the hydrogen bond donor and acceptor indices are obtained from a rule-based method derived from experimental values. Similarity indices were calculated using Gaussian-type distance dependence between the probe and the atoms of the molecules of the data set. This functional form requires no arbitrary definition of cutoff limits, and the similarity indices can be calculated at all grid points inside and outside the molecule. The value of the attenuation factor was set to 0.30.

3D-QSAR models calculation, internal and external validation

In order to generate statistically significant 3D-QSAR models, Partial Least Square (PLS) regression was used to analyse the training set by correlating the variation in the pI_{50} values (the dependent variable) with variations in their CoMFA/CoMSIA interaction fields (the independent variables). The grid was chosen with resolution of 2 Å and extended beyond the molecular dimensions by 4 Å in all directions. Column filtering was set to 4 kcal/mol. CoMFA and CoMSIA models were developed using the conventional stepwise procedure. The leave-one-out cross validation (LOO-CV) was performed to determine optimum number of component leading to the highest cross-validated coefficient q^2 (equation 1) and the lowest standard error of prediction (SEP) that indicates the consistency and predictive ability of models. After that, non-cross-validation was performed to derive the final PLS regressions models with the explained variance r^2, standard error of estimate (S) and F ratio. S represents the measure of the target property uncertainty still unexplained after the model has been derived, and F the ratio of r^2 to 1- r^2 weighted so that the fewer the explanatory properties and more the values of the target property, the higher the F-ratio.

$$q^2 = 1 - \frac{\sum_y \left(Y_{predict} - Y_{experimental}\right)^2}{\sum_y \left(Y_{experimental} - Y_{mean}\right)^2} \qquad (1)$$

Where:

- $Y_{predict}$ = a predicted pI_{50}
- $Y_{experimental}$ = an experimental pI_{50}
- Y_{mean} = the best estimate of the mean of all values that might be predicted
- The numerator is the sum of the squared deviations between predicted and experimental pI_{50} values for the training set compounds.
- The denominator is the sum of the squared deviation between the experimental pI_{50} values and the mean pI_{50} predicted value of the training set

As the name suggests, leave-one-out cross-validation involves using a single observation from the original sample as the validation data, and the remaining observations as the training data. The coefficients of the independent variables of the original PLS model are calculated, excluding one compound (i.e., activity values and calculated properties) from the original training set at once, and this "new" model is used to predict the activity of the excluded compound. This procedure is repeated through the whole data set, until all compounds have been excluded once, and then, q^2 values and SEP are calculated.

The CoMFA/CoMSIA results were graphically represented by field contour maps, where the coefficients were generated using the field type "Stdev*Coeff". Favored and disfavored levels were fixed at 80% and 20%, respectively.

The models generated have to be validated. Even if the model is validated as high quality by internal cross validation, uncertainty will remain regarding its ability to predict chemicals not in the training set. To address this question, external validation data sets are used.

External validation

In order to assess the actual predictive ability of the best models generated by the CoMFA/CoMSIA approaches, the pI_{50} values of the external validation set (i.e., test set compounds not included in the training set) were calculated using the same CoMFA/CoMSIA parameters as those used to generate the models. The non cross validated analyses were used to make predictions of the percent inhibitions of the betulin derivatives compounds from the test set and to display the coefficient contour maps. The actual versus predicted percent inhibitions of the test betulin derivatives compounds were fitted by linear regression, and the "predictive" r^2, S, and F ratio were determined. The quality of the external prediction is documented using the standard deviation of error prediction (r^2 pred).

$$r^2_{pred} = 1 - \frac{\text{PRESS}}{\text{SD}} \tag{2}$$

In Equation (2), PRESS is the sum of the squared deviations between predicted and actual pI_{50} values for the test set compounds and SD is the sum of the squared deviation between the actual pI_{50} values of the compounds from the test set and the mean pI_{50} value of the training set compounds.

Establishing an applicability domain is a major step in QSAR analysis since an applicability domain allows to avoid trying to predict irrelevant molecules, i.e. molecules that differ too much from those included in the training set.(Tropsha, 2010) We have verified that several statistical criteria from activity/property of training and test set prediction defined by Tropsha and al are satisfied by our predictive model, including a correlation coefficient > 0.50, coefficient of determination > 0.60.(Tropsha & Golbraikh, 2007)

2.4 Pharmacophore models

In this study, five compounds from the training set, whose functional R groups are matching well the molecular fields suggested by the CoMFA or CoMSIA models to be important for activity, were selected to generate pharmacophore models: compounds 4, 18, 21, 24 and 25. In the case of the present study, these compounds are also the most active compounds and therefore could have been chosen without the help of the CoMFA/CoMSIA model, but this is not always the case. GALAHAD was run with default values to generate a set of pharmacophore models, used for screening, and molecular alignments, that we do not further use.

GALAHAD is a proprietary pharmacophore module from Tripos Ldt, which generates pharmacophore models and alignments from sets of compounds (Tripos International, St. Louis). A pharmacophore model consist of a group of features located relatively close one to each other in 3D space, surrounded by a sphere of tolerance, which encode location-dependent chemical characteristics that account for activity. The sphere represents the 3D area that should be occupied by specific chemical functional groups for optimal activity. GALAHAD identifies a set of molecular conformations with an optimal combination of low strain energy, steric overlap, and pharmacophoric similarity. The search of conformations is performed in two steps. First, the ligands are aligned one onto each other in internal coordinate space. In this stage a genetic algorithm is used to identify a set of ligand conformations that both minimizes energy and maximizes pharmacosteric similarity. Simultaneously, pharmacophore multiplet similarity between ligands is maximized. This stage is fully flexible. The second step is a rigid-body hypermolecular alignment process in Cartesian space.(Richmond et al., 2004) GALAHAD uses a multi-objective (MO) function in which each term is considered independently for three different purposes: to assess reproductive fitness, to pick the candidates that survive to the next generation, and to rank models after Cartesian alignment of their constituent ligand conformers.(Gillet et al., 2002) The three MO functions (multi-objective triage approach) make use of Pareto ranking for each individual model, which is defined as the number of alternative candidates that are better than the model being assessed by all criteria. (Clark & Abrahamian,). Among the selected models, the ones with the best energy, steric and pharmacophoric concordance values based on Pareto ranking were selected as the best model.

2.5 Database searching and compound selecting

Database searching and compounds selection from the resulting 3D pharmacophore models was carried out on a Linux Pentium (2 CPUs). The private FIMM library (119027 compounds) of Institute for Molecular Medicine Finland and the public NCI library (234054 compounds) of National Cancer Institute were chosen for virtual screening; compounds from these libraries are easily accessible to us for experimental testing. All compounds in these databases were first converted from 2D (sdf format) to 3D using the Concord module in Sybyl-X, and one representative 3D conformation, (lowest energy) selected. Then, for all of these representative conformations, Gasteiger-Huckel charges were assigned and the compounds energy minimized using the standard Tripos force field (Powell method and 0.05 kcal/(mol.Å) energy gradient convergence criteria).

A 3D query was defined based on the best 3D pharmacophore model derived by GALAHAD in Sybyl-X. The query was used to perform virtual screening experiment, by using the Unity 3D database search protocol with all options set to default. In the default option, in order to save screening and hit selection time, the oral bioavailability drug-likeness rule (Lipinski's rule of five with one violation) was applied as a pre-filter with following criterion: molecular weight < 500, -4 < *logp* < 5, number of donor/acceptor < 10, the numbers of rotable bond < 10 and the number of rotatable bonds < 10. This should be also beneficial for the quality of selected compounds at the end of screening.

During the Unity search procedure, the conformations of the compounds in the screened database were generated on the fly by means of the Directed Tweak method.(Hurst, 1994) This procedure attempts to determine if a candidate structure can reasonably flex into a conformation that matches the query. In this way, the data storage problem and the search time are minimized, since only the relevant conformations are dynamically generated. If the query uses spatial constraints, then the query is aligned to the target values for the constraints. If the query contains normal constraints, then the query is aligned to the target for the features. As a result, two hit lists were generated, one for the FIMM and one for the NCI library, which contain compounds with chemical functionalities and spatial properties similar to those of the 3D pharmacophore query. For each compound, a fit value was returned that represented how well the compound fit into the pharmacophore model. The molecular conformations that have been identified by UNITY as hits are not necessarily the lowest possible energy conformations. In some cases, UNITY returns highly strained conformations that energetically cannot exist. The post-processing ranking, relaxing, and tightening functionality allows to rank the hits after the search. In addition, predicted values of the inhibition (I_{50}) percentage and the water-octanol partition coefficients LogP for each compound in the hit lists are computed with CoMSIA predictive model and the Sybyl-X software respectively. LogP is linked to solubility and we may encounter experimental problems to solubilize these compounds. In addition, betulin derivatives are exetrmily hydrophobic and not too much drug-like, where a logP <5 or often < 3 are recommended. Nonetheless, previous studies on betulin have shown it has other advantages that make this scaffold attractive to medicinal chemists.

3. Results and discussion

3.1 3D-QSAR results

CoMFA/CoMSIA modeling and outlier removal

The Fig. 1 shows how the training set molecules are aligned within the grid box (grid spacing 2 A°). The summary of results from CoMFA and CoMSIA models using LOO-CV is presented in Table 2. The predictability of the models is one of the most important parameters for appreciation of 3D-QSAR methods. The first CoMFA/CoMSIA model generated with all compounds in the training set has a Q^2 value of 0.27 and 0.30 respectively. The analysis of correlations between the calculated and experimental values of pI_{50} (Fig. 2) show the presence of two compounds, 6 and 12, poorly predicted. Compounds 6 and 12 are at extreme of experimental property/activity range from all others values: compound 6 is inactive and compound 12 is highly active. In addition, these compounds carry strong electrophilic centers that are good leaving groups (compounds 12) or Michael acceptors (compound 6). It is likely that the bioactivities of these compounds are due to their high reactivity, i.e. their tendencies to covalently attach to nucelophilic centers. In order to avoid mixing up different mechanistic effects, the CoMFA/CoMSIA models were rebuilt omitting these compounds, considering them as outliers. Compound 16, which present similarly to compound 12 a good leaving group, was accordingly deleted from the test set. On the other hand, compounds 4 and 22, which contain potentially reactive aldehydes in their substituent, were kept in the dataset since aldehydes are not very reactive groups and can be found in known drugs.

CoMFA model, predictivity

As a result, the CoMFA model without compounds 6 and 12 describing Betulin derivatives inhibition used both steric and electrostatic fields and had a Q^2 value of 0.58, and using two components. This CoMFA model indicated different contributions of both steric and electrostatic fields of 0.33 and 0.66, respectively. The model had cross-validated $r^2 = 0.58$, non cross-validated $r^2 = 0.81$ and Fischer ratio ($F = 24.11$). The predictions of pI_{50} values for the 14 BDIs in the training set using CoMFA models are shown in Table 1. The correlations between the calculated and experimental values of pI_{50} (from training and LOO cross-validation) are shown in Fig. 2.

This model was validated by an external test set of eight compounds not included in the model construction. We found that this model was able to describe the test set variance with predictive r^2 = 0.78. The predicted activity values of test set are listed in Table 1, and the correlations between the predictions and experimental values are represented in Fig. 2. This analysis revealed that the proposed model is able to predict successfully compounds that were not used in the training process.

CoMFA model, contour plots

The contour plots of the CoMFA steric and electrostatic fields are presented in Fig. 3 for the modeled BDI activities. For simplicity, only the most active compound (compound 18) contour map is shown. In this figure, green and yellow contours indicate regions where steric bulk groups favored and disfavored the activity, respectively. A green contour, shown in Fig. 3, indicates that large substituents near C2 of the compound 18 (substituent R1) are important for a high BD inhibitory activity. The red contours at the same position indicate regions where an increase of positive charge decreases the activity. The R1 substituents are therefore preferably large and negatively charged. Green contours are also located near the R2 substituent at C16 (Fig. 3) that therefore prefers large substituents too. Overall, polar groups are favored at R2. Red contours indicate that functional groups containing with an electronegative character, such as carboxylic acid (COO-) and OH, are beneficial at R2. Positively charged groups, such as bases and OH groups, are also beneficial at R2 for gaining BDI activity, as seen by the blue contours. It seems that the R3 substitution does not have any effect on compound activity according the steric and electrostatic field contours, but as mentioned before the conformational alignment of this substituent was not optimized.

CoMSIA model, predictivity

In comparison to CoMFA, CoMSIA is less affected by changes in molecular alignment and provides smoother and interpretable contour maps as a result of employing Gaussian type distance dependence with the molecular similarity indices it uses. Furthermore, in addition to the steric and electrostatic fields, CoMSIA defines explicit hydrophobic and HBD and HBA descriptor fields. A more statistically robust model was obtained from the CoMSIA study. The CoMSIA model has a better cross-validated r^2 value of 0.662 using five components, non cross-validated r^2 value of 0.991 and a Fischer ratio (F = 179.83). CoMSIA model indicated contributions of steric, electrostatic, hydrophobic, H bonds donor and acceptor field contributions of 0.03, 0.31, 0.07, 0.34 and 0.22 respectively. Thus, in contrast to CoMFA, the steric contribution to the CoMSIA model is almost neglictible. The predictions of pI_{50} values for the 14 BDIs in the training set using CoMSIA model are shown in Table 1. The correlations between the calculated and experimental values of pI_{50} (from training and LOO-CV are shown in Fig. 4. The CoMSIA model was also used to predict the inhibitory activities of the external test set compounds, and this model was able to describe the test set with predictive r^2 = 0.91. The external test set predicted values are listed in Table 1, and the correlations between the predicted activity values and experimental values are represented in Fig. 4. As for CoMFA, the model is therefore able to predict successfully compounds that were not used in the training process.

CoMSIA model, contour plots

The contour plots of the CoMSIA steric, electrostatic, hydrophobic, HB acceptor and HB donor fields are presented in Fig. 5. Generally, the steric and electrostatic field contributions respectively are similar to those one in CoMFA analysis (Fig. 5a). They were interpreted in the same manner as in the above-mentioned CoMFA model and therefore not described here.

CoMSIA models present, in addition to CoMFA models, hydrophobic and hydrogen-bond fields. The hydrophobic contributions are presented in Fig. 5b. An orange contour covering the area near substituent R2 indicates that hydrophobic groups are favoured at R2. Instead, the presence of black contours at R1 substitution, near C3, suggests that hydrophilic groups are useful to increase activity. The hydrogen bond donor and acceptors contours are generally in agreement with the contours based on negative/positive charges, as seen on Fig. 5c and 4d, however giving more precise information. A large magenta contour near R2 shows that HB donor groups are favourable to activity at R2. A significant volume red contour is present near to C16 indicates a detrimental effect of HB acceptor groups at R1, an information that was not given by the CoMFA model. Red contour near the R1 substituent, that hydrogen bond acceptor groups at R1 decrease the activity.

Performance comparison

The superior performance of CoMSIA relative to CoMFA with this dataset may be attributed to the smoother potentials or to the higher contributions from the HBD and HBA fields to the CoMSIA models (Table 2). Unlike CoMSIA, CoMFA does not have explicit hydrogen-bonding descriptors, which are assumed to be implicitly treated in the CoMFA steric and electrostatic fields, respectively. The CoMSIA steric and electrostatic PLS contours were similarly placed as those of the CoMFA model. The HBD fields made the highest contribution to the CoMSIA models (Table 2), which suggest that among the descriptors considered, the HBD is the most important factor influencing the activity of the betulin derivatives in the training set.

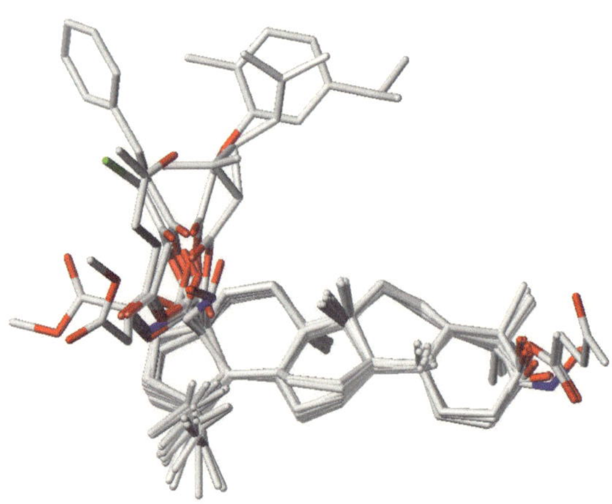

Fig. 1. Database alignment superposition of training set compounds used for 3D-QSAR analysis

	Parameter						Contributions				
	r^2_{cv}	NC	r^2_{ncv}	SEE	*F*-value	r^2_{pred}	S	E	H	D	A
CoMFA	0.27	1	-	-	-	-	-	-	-	-	-
CoMSIA	0.30	2	-	-	-	-	-	-	-	-	-
CoMFA*	0.58	2	0.81	0.44	24.11	0.78	0.33	0.66	-	-	-
CoMSIA*	0.66	5	0.99	0.11	179.83	0.91	0.03	0.31	0.07	0.34	0.22

Table 2. Summary of Analysis Results of the CoMFA and CoMSIA Models. NC is the number of components from PLS analysis, r^2_{cv} are the correlation coefficients of the leave-one-out (LOO) cross-validation, r^2_{ncv} are the correlation coefficients for training set without cross-validation analysis. S = Steric, E = Electrostatic, H = Hydrophobic, D = H bond donor, A = H bond acceptor

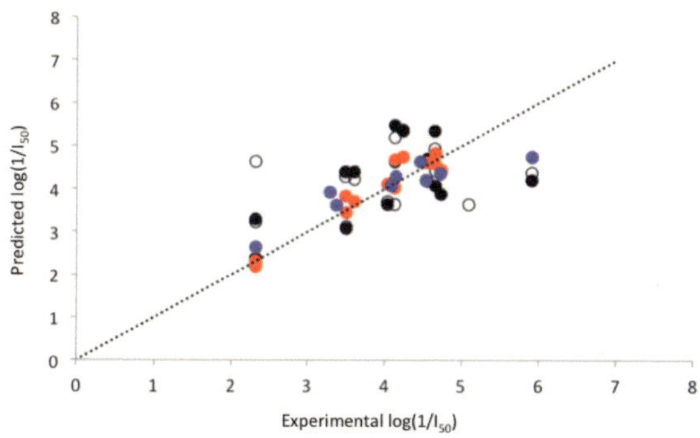

Fig. 2. Scatter plot of the experimental activities versus predicted activities for the CoMFA model. Empty circles: LOO cross-validated predictions on the full training set. Black circles: LOO cross-validated predictions on training set predictions without compound 6 and 12. Red circles: training set without cross validation, Blue circle: test-set predictions.

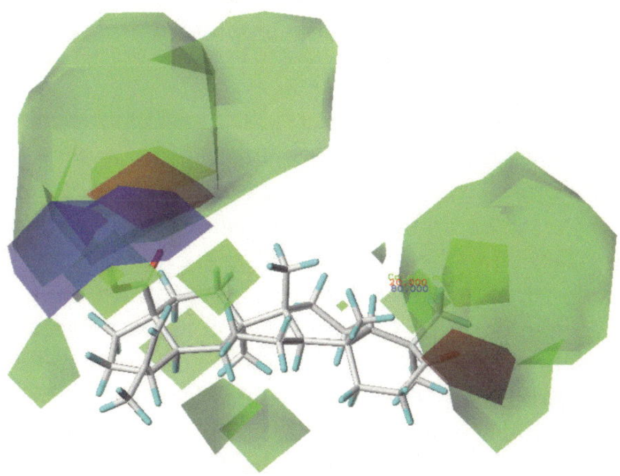

Fig. 3. Contour maps for CoMFA with compound 18 shown as a representative structure. Green contours indicate regions where bulky groups enhance the activity. Blue contours indicate regions where an increase of positive charge enhances the activity, and red contours indicate regions where more negative charges are favourable for activity.

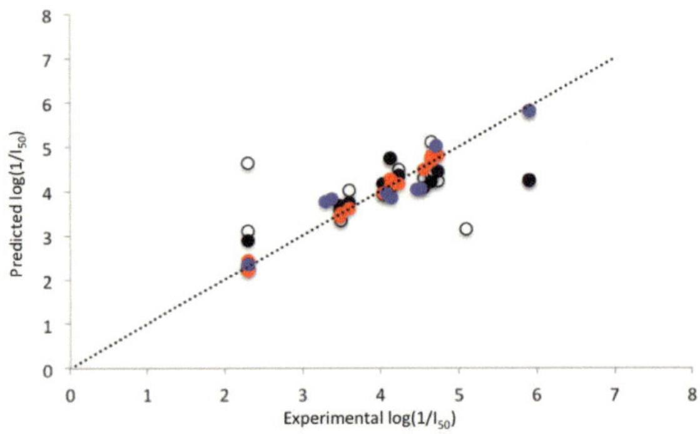

Fig. 4. Scatter plot of the experimental activities versus predicted activities for CoMSIA model. Empty circles: LOO cross-validated predictions on full training set, Black circles: LOO cross-validated predictions on training set predictions without compound 6 and 12, Red circles: training set without cross validation, Blue circles: test-set predictions.

3.2 Pharmacophoric representations

GALAHAD pharmacophore models were derived, by using the 5 most active ligands in the training set (these 5 compounds are shown in bold in Table 1). Ten pharmacophore models were retained after the GALAHAD runs. All these models present eight to nine pharmacophoric features. Seven hydrophobic moieties of the pharmacophore reflect the presence for a large hydrophobic structure as the skeleton of the BDIs. It would be possible for us to reduce the number of these pharmacophoric points if we wished to retrieve chemical compounds more distant from the betulin scaffold. The remaining 2 to 3 pharmacophoric points corresponds to the three R groups. In Fig. 7, the pharmacophore for model 3 is represented. It includes 8 pharmacophore features: 7 hydrophobes (HY_2, HY_3, HY_4, HY_5, HY_6, HY_7 and HY_8) and 1 HD donors (DA_1). The HB donor moieties reflect the importance of OH groups at these positions of the betulin for BD inhibitory activity. In Fig. 7, cyan and magenta spheres represent indicate hydrophobes and HB donors, respectively.

Each of the obtained models represents a different trade-off among the conflicting demands of maximizing steric consensus, maximizing pharmacophore consensus, and minimizing energy. They had Pareto rank 0; this means no one model is superior to any other. During GALAHAD runs, it is recognized that high-energy values are due to steric clashes.(Dorfman et al., 2008) The algorithm retains these models to keep good characteristics to be passed on to less strained offspring during genetic algorithm process. All the GALAHAD models are derived from at least 4 ligands of the training set and were compared according to Pareto ranking. Table 3 shows energy, steric and pharmacophoric concordance values for models with all the 5 ligands. Minimum and maximum values for each characteristic between all the obtained twenty models are also reported in this table. The model ten had energy very high than the other nine models and is not included in the statistic. Small value of energy and high values of steric and pharmacophoric concordance are desired for the best model. Now, the higher energy value between all the models is 6149; the models containing all the five ligands had values between 41.79 (the minimum) and 6149.39 (the maximum), in this sense energy value varies widely distributed among the considered models. Steric had a small

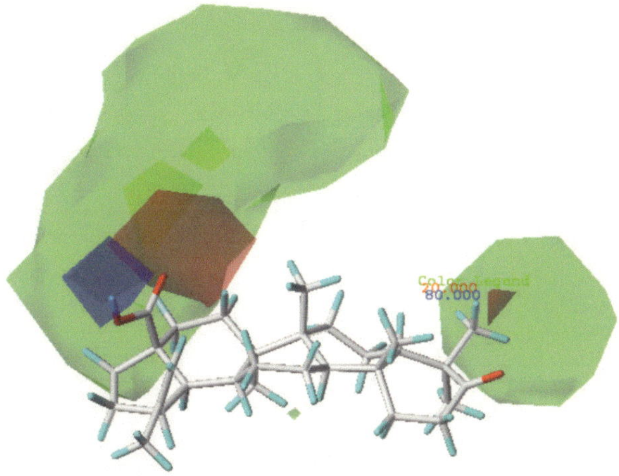
20.000
80.000

(A)

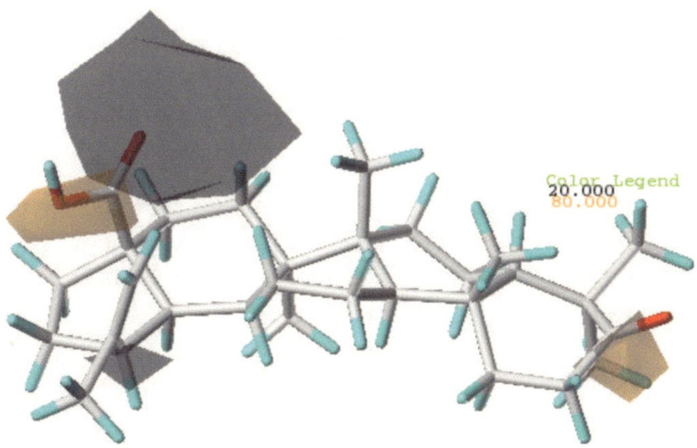
Color Legend
20.000
80.000

(B)

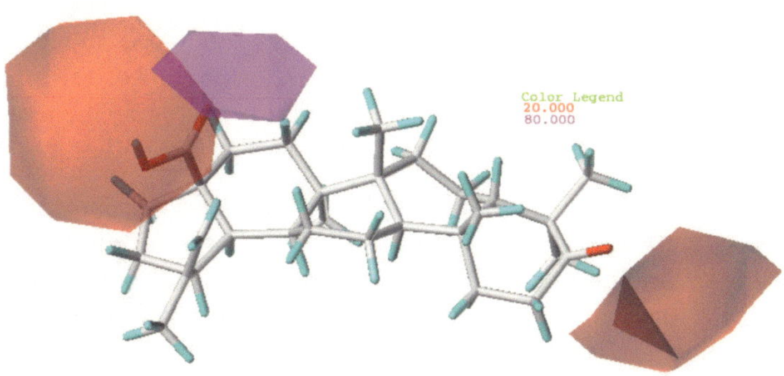
Color Legend
20.000
80.000

(C)

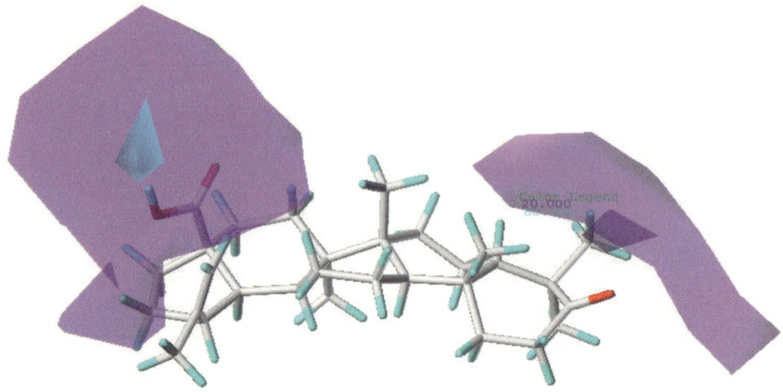

(D)

Fig. 5. Contour maps for the CoMSIA model, shown with compound 18 as a representative structure. (A) Steric field: green contours indicates region where bulky groups enhance the activity. Electrostatic field: Blue indicates regions where positive charge is favoured and enhances activity and red the regions where it decrease it. (B) Hydrophobic field: orange contours indicate regions where hydrophobic/hydrophilic groups enhance/decrease the activity, and black contours indicate regions where hydrophobic/hydrophilic groups decrease/enhance the activity. (C) HB acceptor field: Magenta represents areas where HB acceptors favor the activity and red, area where it disfavour it. (D) HB donor field: Cyan represents areas where HB donors favor the activity and purple the area where it decrease it.

variation between the minimum (20978.80) and the maximum (21538.59) considering all the models. Finally, pharmacophoric concordance had a small variation between the minimum (325) and the maximum (392.50). With the intention to select the best model, we constructed a 3D plot to visualize the Pareto surface (Fig. 6).

Considering only the energy and steric criteria, the best of all models lies in the upper left hand corner of the graph in Fig. 6a, where the energy (x axis) is low and the steric (y axis) score is high. In terms of pharmacophoric concordance and steric criteria, the best of all models lies in the upper right hand corner of the graph in Fig. 6b, where the HBond (x axis) score is high and steric (y axis) is high. Finally, in terms of pharmacophoric concordance and energy scores, the best of all models now lies at the lower right corner, where HBOND (x axis) are high and energy (y axis) are low both (Fig. 6c). According Fig. 6, there is only one model (Model 3), which filled all the three requirements described above and was selected for the next of study. This model is represented in Fig. 7. Model 3 has low energy, the higher steric but with high pharmacophoric concordance values. All conformers aligned represent low-energy conformations of the molecules, and it can be seen that the final alignment shows a satisfactory superimposition of the pharmacophoric points.

We evaluated how well the model identifies active compounds in virtual screening experiment of a larger database. For this, the model was used to screen a large database constituted by FIMM database, NCI database and the set of 24 compounds from the previous 3D-QSAR studies. This indicates how these models can be used as a theoretical screening tool and how they were able to discriminate between active and inactive molecules, and consequently, to predict whether a new molecule inhibits BD.

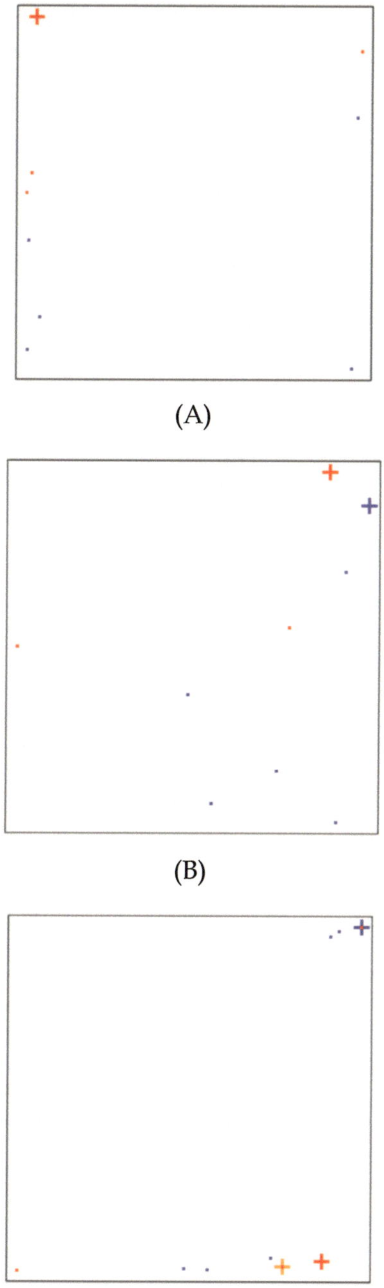

(A)

(B)

(C)

Fig. 6. Plot of the strain energy, steric overlap and pharmacophoric concordance values for GALAHAD models with all the 5 ligands with contribution to the consensus feature.

Plot of steric overlap vs. energy. (B) Plot of steric overlap vs. pharmacophoric concordance (HBOND). (C) Plot of HBOND vs. steric overlap.

MODEL	Features	ENERGY	STERICS	HBOND
MODEL 1	9	6074.6299	21377.9004	388.1
MODEL 2	8	41.79	21258.1992	325
MODEL 3	**8**	**210.97**	**21538.5996**	**385.1**
MODEL 4	9	75.67	21181.9004	357.9
MODEL 5	8	126.38	21289.6992	377.3
MODEL 6	9	5978.9502	20978.8008	386.4
MODEL 7	9	279.49	21061.1992	375
MODEL 8	9	56.97	21009	362.5
MODEL 9	8	6149.3901	21483.5	392.5
MODEL 10	9	132872792	21596.6992	366
Min[a]		41.79	20978.8008	325
Max[a]		6149.3901	21538.5996	392.5

Table 3. Summary of Analysis Results of the CoMFA and CoMSIA Models. The selected model (MODEL 3) is indicated in boldface. [a]Minimum and maximum values between all the obtained 21 models.

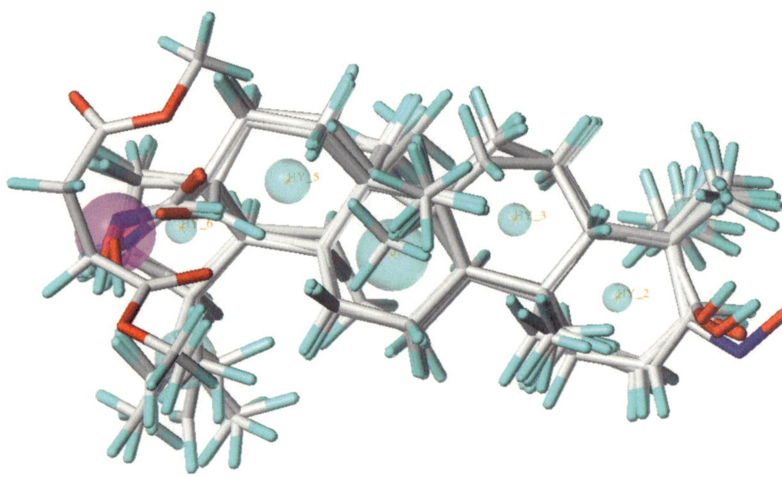

Fig. 7. Selected pharmacophore model 3 and molecular alignment of the compounds used to elaborate the models. Cyan, and magenta spheres are represented for hydrophobes, and HB donors, respectively.

3.3 Virtual screening results

Before screening a virtual database it is important to verify the (dis)similarity of compounds present in the database. This enables us to visualize the chemical space covered by the compounds inside the database and the level of diversity of these compounds. The diversity of a library of compounds denotes the degree of heterogeneity, structural range within the set of compounds. Such exploration of yet unknown chemical space might help to solve the problem of the high attrition rates in drug development by giving more diverse compounds to choose, a broader range of structures at the hit prioritization level, which should increase the chances of success at later stages and also may allow us to avoid target promiscuity that is apparent in many drugs and allow the design of safer drugs. The chemical space of chemical (diversity/similarity) of chemical structure libraries can be characterized by the distribution of Tanimoto coefficients (equation 3). The Tanimoto coefficient is the most commonly used coefficient in chemical similarity/diversity work, following a study of the performance of a range of similarity coefficients by Willet and Winterman.(Willett & Winterman, 1986) It firstly requires that the molecules are represented by appropriate structural descriptors. Many different structural descriptors have been developed for similarity searching in chemical databases including 2D fragment based descriptors, 3D descriptors, and descriptors that are based on the physical properties of molecules.(Downs et al., 1994) The Tanimoto coefficient is usually calculated from the 2D structure fingerprint, or the 3D shape/feature similarity. A fingerprint is an ordered list of bits. Each bit represents a Boolean determination of, or test for, the presence of, for example, an element count, a type of ring system, atom pairing, atom environment (nearest neighbors), etc., in a chemical structure.

The Tanimoto score equation:

$$T(A,B) = \frac{AB}{\|A\|^2 + \|B\|^2 - AB} \tag{3}$$

Where:
T(A,B) is the similarity score, a fraction between 0 and 1.
A is the count of bits set in fingerprint A
B is the count of bits set in fingerprint B
AB is the count of bits set in common in fingerprints A and B

The Unity module generates a binary substructure fingerprint for chemical structures of our screening libraries. These fingerprints are used by Unity for similarity neighboring and similarity searching. As shown in Fig. 8 and Fig. 9, when we calculated the matrix of pairwise similarity based on 2D structure for the FIMM and NCI libraries. This 2D fingerprints is based on a combination of a hashing function (which represents connected molecular fragments in a efficient but unintelligible manner) and an explicit count of specific fragments, such as rings. The histograms of the Tanimoto indices show diverse distribution of the compounds in the databases and relative distribution of type of compounds inside. A 2D Tanimoto mean of 0.88 and 0.87 are indicative of a suitable range of diversity within each of the two databases.

The Model shown in Fig. 7 was used to generate the query for 3D search virtual screening via the 3D search method implemented in UNITY module encoded in Tripos. Compounds had to map at least 6 features in the pharmacophore model.

```
<<
DONOR_ATOM[NAME=DA_1;TARGET=(-6.205,0.423,2.026)]
HYDROPHOBIC[NAME=HY_2;TARGET=(3.520,-0.863,-0.432)]
HYDROPHOBIC[NAME=HY_3;TARGET=(1.540,0.665,0.009)]
HYDROPHOBIC[NAME=HY_4;TARGET=(-0.820,-0.017,-0.450)]
HYDROPHOBIC[NAME=HY_5;TARGET=(-2.846,1.434,-0.588)]
HYDROPHOBIC[NAME=HY_6;TARGET=(-4.916,0.526,-1.145)]
HYDROPHOBIC[NAME=HY_7;TARGET=(4.890,0.689,-0.736)]
```

```
HYDROPHOBIC[NAME=HY_8;TARGET=(-4.841,-2.039,-0.846)]
spatial_point[name=SPAT_DA_1;feature=DA_1;point=(-6.205,0.423,2.026);tolerance=0.800]
spatial_point[name=SPAT_HY_2;feature=HY_2;point=(3.520,-0.863,-0.432);tolerance=0.290]
spatial_point[name=SPAT_HY_3;feature=HY_3;point=(1.540,0.665,0.009);tolerance=0.330]
spatial_point[name=SPAT_HY_4;feature=HY_4;point=(-0.820,-0.017,-0.450);tolerance=0.710]
spatial_point[name=SPAT_HY_5;feature=HY_5;point=(-2.846,1.434,-0.588);tolerance=0.450]
spatial_point[name=SPAT_HY_6;feature=HY_6;point=(-4.916,0.526,-1.145);tolerance=0.310]
spatial_point[name=SPAT_HY_7;feature=HY_7;point=(4.890,0.689,-0.736);tolerance=0.410]
spatial_point[name=SPAT_HY_8;feature=HY_8;point=(-4.841,-2.039,-0.846);tolerance=0.600]
partial_match[min=6;max=6;features=DA_1,HY_2,HY_3,HY_4,HY_5,HY_6,HY_7,HY_8]
>>
```

As a result (see Table 4), pharmacophore based virtual screening yielded 13 hits (out of 24) from Table 1 compounds, 16 hits from FIMM library (out of 120k compounds) and 76 hits from NCI library (out of 240k compounds) that meet the specified requirements. The hits list selected from the Table 1 compounds confirm the selectivity of our query. Among the set of 24 betulin derivatives used as controls, about half (13) were retrieved by the procedure, mostly the highly active ones. Finally, as a result of this study the best 20 hits from FIMM and NCI were selected for further pharmacological assay (Table 5 and 6). The inhibition (I_{50}) percentage of the selected compounds are in the range of the values of active compounds present in the Table 1 dataset and their values of LogP are near the value (8.07) of the most active compound (compound 18) of Table 1. These predicted values of I_{50} and LogP should be used to prioritize compounds to send in experimental test.

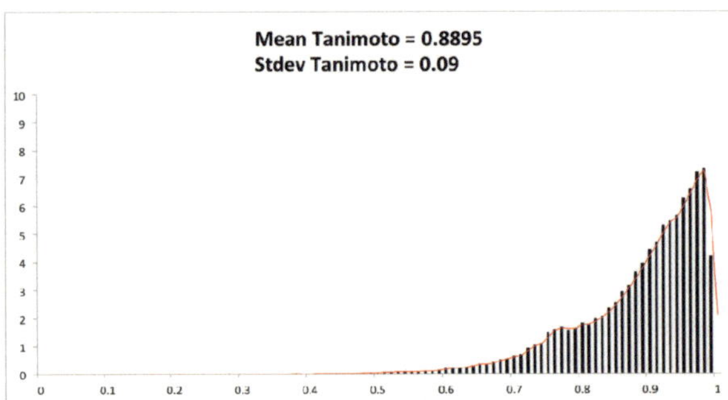

Fig. 8. FIMM library distribution

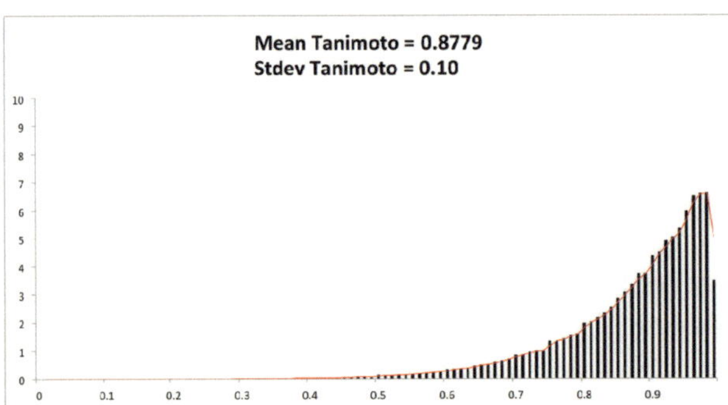

Fig. 9. NCI library distribution

	Table 1	FIMM	NCI
Number hits	13	16	76

Table 4. Summary of hits found by pharmacophore based 3D search virtual screening on FIMM, NCI and table 1 compound.

FIMM ID	Image	QFIT	RANK	LOGBIO	CLOGP
538990053	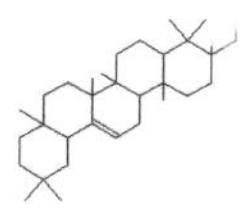	34.33	1	3.63	10.66
538990110	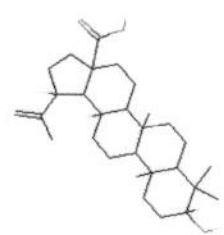	22.94	2	3.66	7.95
538990111	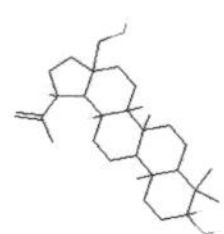	27.42	3	3.67	8.52
538990154	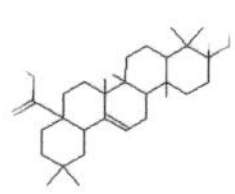	34.33	4	3.69	8.62
538990271	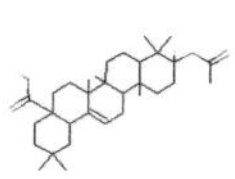	34.33	5	3.52	9.53
538990190	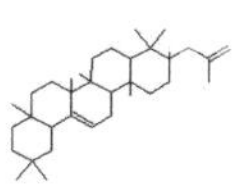	34.33	6	3.39	11.60
538990189	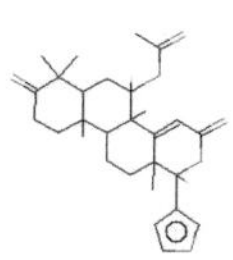	46.28	7	4.37	3.88

538990181	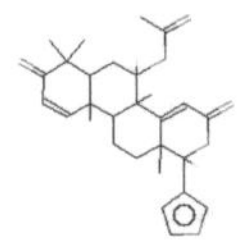	35.60	8	4.25	3.74
538990200	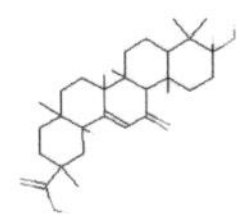	39.75	9	3.67	6.47
538990295	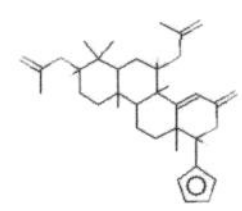	45.39	10	4.00	5.23
AE-641/00404032	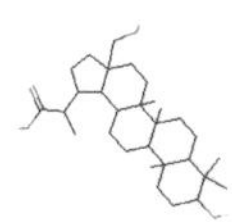	56.28	11	3.76	6.97
538990112	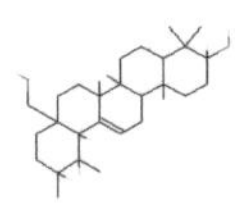	47.15	12	3.66	8.67
538988558	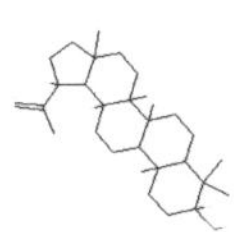	56.28	13	3.55	10.51
538990155	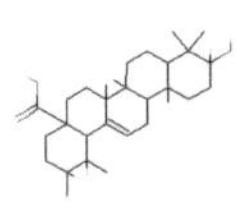	47.15	14	3.73	8.62
538990368	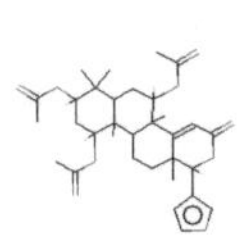	42.53	15	3.68	4.67
538990294	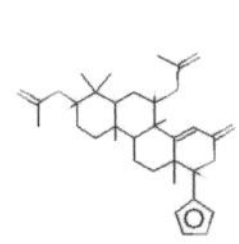	45.39	16	4.07	5.23

Table 5. List of compounds selected with pharmacophore based 3D search virtual screening on FIMM compounds.

NCI ID	Image	QFIT	RANK	LOGBIO	CLOGP
661747	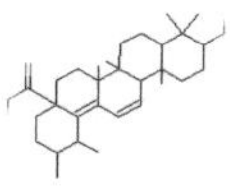	80.42	1	3.55	8.40
144946	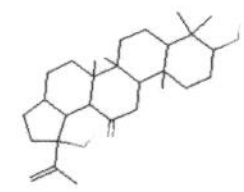	64.10	2	3.70	6.14
680072	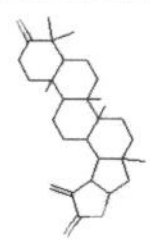	30.81	3	3.68	7.07
152534	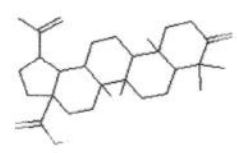	30.60	4	3.81	8.075
250423	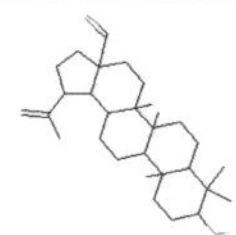	60.03	5	3.70	8.44
277277	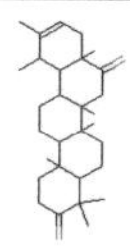	30.62	6	4.06	7.77
119118	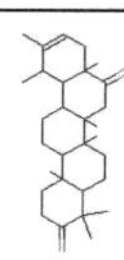	30.62	7	4.06	7.77
527971	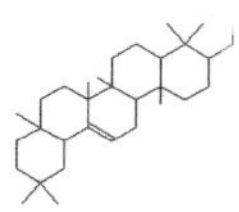	53.78	8	3.70	10.66
90487	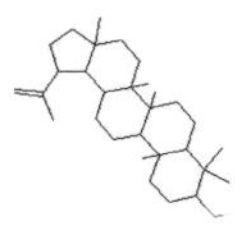	60.03	9	3.68	10.51
152535	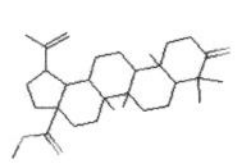	30.60	10	3.83	8.45
403166	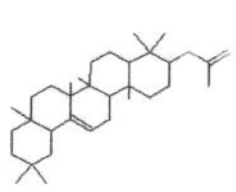	53.78	11	3.59	11.60

281807	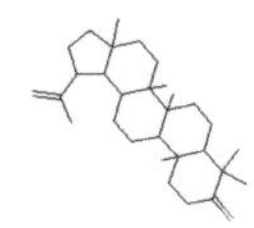	20.53	12	3.82	10.11
114945	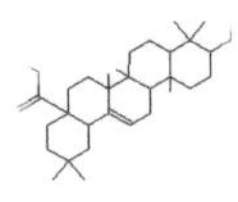	53.78	13	3.70	8.62
113090	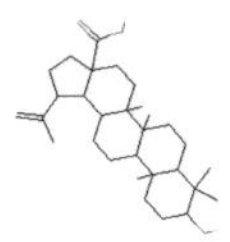	60.03	14	3.70	8.47
655415	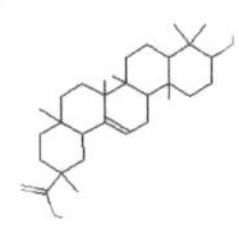	53.78	15	3.67	8.62
94656	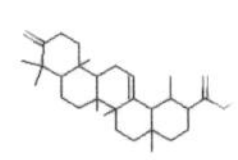	50.21	16	3.93	8.22
655414	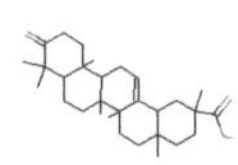	50.21	17	3.81	8.22
125854	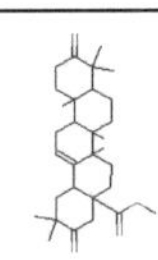	51.71	18	3.91	6.86
677578	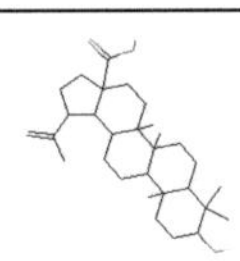	60.03	19	3.70	8.47
133914	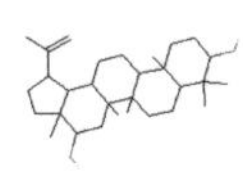	29.32	20	3.63	8.42

Table 6. List of compounds selected with pharmacophore based 3D search virtual screening on NCI compounds.

4. Conclusions

In the current study, 3D-QSAR and pharmacophore models were derived for betulin derivatives as inhibitors of Leishmaniases, which should be useful for assisting the design of active compounds. Such models correlate well structural features with inhibitory activities and bring valuable information about the relevant characteristics of inhibitors. CoMFA and CoMSIA approaches were developed to derive structure-activity relationships. CoMFA and

CoMSIA modeling were efficients tools to suggest outliers that we could link to a specific molecular mechanism, in that case covalent crosslinking. The models are reliable and were obtained by using steric and electrostatic CoMFA fields, and by using steric, electrostatic, hydrophobic, HB acceptor and donor CoMSIA fields. In this study, CoMSIA outperforms CoMFA, but this is not always the case. Moreover, contour plots may help identify relevant regions where any change can affect binding preference. According to the obtained statistics, prediction of betulin derivatives activities with sufficient accuracy should be possible by using these models. In a second phase, pharmacophore models were derived with GALAHAD. Models derived from 5 active compounds that all match best the CoMSIA predictions were obtained. These models include hydrophobes, and HB donors. The obtained pharmacophore models were used as queries for 3D flexible search engine to search for the FIMM, NCI and QSAR dataset collection. Without the verification of the predictive characteristic of the compounds in our dataset with 3D-QSAR model, it would have been much more speculative to do a pharmacophore-based screening. The process of screening takes less than two hours (standard 2 CPUs workstation). In comparison, a molecular docking study involving the same two libraries in the same conditions, counting 2-5 seconds (2 CPU) for each compound, would take 20 to 50 hours. The search was really efficient, allowing us to retrieve among the hit lists 9 out of the 14 molecules that had been used to build the model and had been put in the library as a control, as well as 4 out of 8 molecules in the test set also used as a control. As a result of this study, 20 first molecules were selected from FIMM and NCI hit list for further biological binding assay.

While this study is conducted for a small number of compounds, for which biological activity was easily obtainable and testing conducted in a single laboratory, it could easily be generalized to larger sets and databases. The results described in this paper indicate that this method is very efficient in the study of hit identification and lead optimization.

5. Acknowledgment

Leo GHEMTIO thanks The Drug Discovery and Chemical Biology Consortium and CDR of University of Helsinki for financial support through a postdoctoral fellowship. Yuezhou Zhang would like to thank the Chinese Scholarship Council for financial support and the Informational and Structural Biology doctoral programme (ISB) for organizing graduate studies. The Finnish IT Center for Science (CSC) is thanked for computational resources.

6. References

Alakurtti, S., Bergström, P., Sacerdoti-Sierra, N., Jaffe, C. L., & Yli-Kauhaluoma, J. (2010) Anti-leishmanial activity of betulin derivatives. J Antibiot (Tokyo) 63, 123-6.

Alakurtti, S., Mäkelä, T., Koskimies, S., & Yli-Kauhaluoma, J. (2006) Pharmacological properties of the ubiquitous natural product betulin. Eur J Pharm Sci 29, 1-13.

Bostrom, J., Bohm, M., Gundertofte, K., & Klebe, G. (2003) A 3D QSAR Study on a Set of Dopamine D₄ Receptor Antagonists. J. Chem. Inf. Comput. Sci. 43, 1020--1027.

Buolamwini, J. K. & Assefa, H. (2003) Overview of Novel Anticancer Drug Targets. 85, .

Clark, R. (2009) Prospective ligand- and target-based 3D QSAR: state of the art 2008.. Current topics in medicinal chemistry 9, 791--810.

Clark, R. D. & Abrahamian, E. () Using a staged multi-objective optimization approach to find selective pharmacophore models. Journal of Computer-Aided Molecular Design 23, 765--771.

Cramer, R., Patterson, D., & Bunce, J. (1988) Comparative molecular field analysis (CoMFA). Effect of shape on binding of steroids to carrier proteins. Journal of the American Chemical Society 110, 5959--5967.

Dorfman, R., Smith, K., Masek, B., & Clark, R. (2008) A knowledge-based approach to generating diverse but energetically representative ensembles of ligand conformers. Journal of Computer-Aided Molecular Design 22, 681-691.

Downs, G. M., Willett, P., & Fisanick, W. (1994) Similarity Searching and Clustering of Chemical-Structure Databases Using Molecular Property Data. Journal of Chemical Information and Computer Sciences 34, 1094-1102.

Ekins, S., Mestres, J., & Testa, B. (2007) In silico pharmacology for drug discovery: applications to targets and beyond.. British journal of pharmacology 152, 21--37.

Ghemtio, L., Devignes, M.-D., Smaïl-Tabbone, M., Souchet, M., Leroux, V., & Maigret, B. (2010) Comparison of Three Preprocessing Filters Efficiency in Virtual Screening: Identification of New Putative LXRβ Regulators As a Test Case. Journal of Chemical Information and Modeling 50, 701-715.

Gillet, V. J., Khatib, W., Willett, P., Fleming, P. J., & Green, D. V. S. (2002) Combinatorial Library Design Using a Multiobjective Genetic Algorithm. Journal of Chemical Information and Computer Sciences 42, 375-385.

Hurst, T. (1994) Flexible 3D searching: The directed tweak technique. Journal of Chemical Information and Computer Sciences 34, 190--196.

Jain, A. N. (2004) Ligand-Based Structural Hypotheses for Virtual Screening. Journal of Medicinal Chemistry 47, 947--961.

Kirchmair, J., Distinto, S., Schuster, D., Spitzer, G., Langer, T., & Wolber, G. (2008) Enhancing Drug Discovery Through In Silico Screening: Strategies to Increase True Positives Retrieval Rates. Current Medicinal Chemistry 15, 2040--2053.

Kirchmair, J., Markt, P., Distinto, S., Wolber, G., & Langer, T. (2008) Evaluation of the performance of 3D virtual screening protocols: RMSD comparisons, enrichment assessments, and decoy selection---What can we learn from earlier mistakes?. Journal of Computer-Aided Molecular Design 22, 213--228.

Klebe, G., Abraham, U., & Mietzner, T. (1994) Molecular Similarity Indices in a Comparative Analysis (CoMSIA) of Drug Molecules to Correlate and Predict Their Biological Activity. Journal of Medicinal Chemistry 37, 4130--4146.

Langer, T. & Hoffmann, R. (2001) Virtual screening: an effective tool for lead structure discovery?. Current pharmaceutical design. 7, 509--527.

Lengauer, T. (2004) Novel technologies for virtual screening. Drug Discovery Today 9, 27--34.

Ling & Xuefeng, B. (2008) High Throughput Screening Informatics. Combinatorial Chemistry & High Throughput Screening 11, 249--257.

Liu, H.-Y., Liu, S.-S., Qin, L.-T., & Mo, L.-Y. () CoMFA and CoMSIA analysis of 2,4-thiazolidinediones derivatives as aldose reductase inhibitors. Journal of Molecular Modeling , .

Nagarajan, S., Ahmed, A., Choo, H., Cho, Y., Oh, K.-S., Lee, B., Shin, K., & Pae, A. (2010) 3D QSAR pharmacophore model based on diverse IKKβ inhibitors. Journal of Molecular Modeling , .

Perkins, R., Fang, H., Tong, W., & Welsh, W. J. (2003) Quantitative structure-activity relationship methods: perspectives on drug discovery and toxicology. Environ Toxicol Chem 22, 1666-79.

Pink, R., Hudson, A., Mouriès, M.-A., & Bendig, M. (2005) Opportunities and challenges in antiparasitic drug discovery. Nat Rev Drug Discov 4, 727-40.

Richmond, N., Abrams, C., Wolohan, P., Abrahamian, E., Willett, P., & Clark, R. (2006) GALAHAD: 1. Pharmacophore identification by hypermolecular alignment of ligands in 3D. Journal of Computer-Aided Molecular Design V20, 567--587.

Richmond, N., Willett, P., & Clark, R. (2004) Alignment of three-dimensional molecules using an image recognition algorithm. Journal of Molecular Graphics and Modelling 23, 199--209.

Rognan, D. (2010) Structure-Based Approaches to Target Fishing and Ligand Profiling. Molecular Informatics 29, 176--187.

Rönkkö, T., Tervo, A., Parkkinen, J., & Poso, A. (2006) BRUTUS: Optimization of a grid-based similarity function for rigid-body molecular superposition. II. Description and characterization. Journal of Computer-Aided Molecular Design 20, 227-236.

Sippl, W. (2002) Development of biologically active compounds by combining 3D QSAR and structure-based design methods.. J Comput Aided Mol Des 16, 825--830.

Spitzer, G., Heiss, M., Mangold, M., Markt, P., Kirchmair, J., Wolber, G., & Liedl, K. (2010) One Concept, Three Implementations of 3D Pharmacophore-Based Virtual Screening: Distinct Coverage of Chemical Search Space.. Journal of chemical information and modeling 0, .

Stahura, F. & Bajorath, J. (2004) Virtual Screening Methods that Complement HTS. Combinatorial Chemistry & High Throughput Screening 7, 259--269.

Tervo, A. J., Rönkkö, T., Nyrönen, T. H., & Poso, A. (2005) BRUTUS: Optimization of a Grid-Based Similarity Function for Rigid-Body Molecular Superposition. 1. Alignment and Virtual Screening Applications. Journal of Medicinal Chemistry 48, 4076--4086.

SYBYL-X 1.2, Tripos International, 1699 South Hanley Rd., St. Louis, Missouri, 63144, USA.

Tropsha, A. (2010) Best Practices for QSAR Model Development, Validation, and Exploitation. Molecular Informatics 29, 476--488.

Tropsha, A. & Golbraikh, A. (2007) Predictive QSAR modeling workflow, model applicability domains, and virtual screening. Current pharmaceutical design 13, 3494--3504.

Tuccinardi, T. (2009) Docking-based virtual screening: recent developments.. Combinatorial chemistry & high throughput screening 12, 303--314.

Vainio, M. J., Puranen, J. S., & Johnson, M. S. (2009) ShaEP: Molecular Overlay Based on Shape and Electrostatic Potential. Journal of Chemical Information and Modeling 49, 492--502.

Villoutreix, B., Eudes, R., & Miteva, M. (2009) Structure-based virtual ligand screening: recent success stories.. Combinatorial chemistry & high throughput screening 12, 1000--1016.

Viswanadhan, V. N., Ghose, A. K., Revankar, G. R., & Robins, R. K. (1989) Atomic physicochemical parameters for three dimensional structure directed quantitative structure-activity relationships. 4. Additional parameters for hydrophobic and dispersive interactions and their application for an automated superposition of certain naturally occurring nucleoside antibiotics. Journal of Chemical Information and Computer Sciences 29, 163-172.

Willett, P. & Winterman, V. (1986) A Comparison of Some Measures for the Determination of Inter-Molecular Structural Similarity Measures of Inter-Molecular Structural Similarity. Quantitative Structure-Activity Relationships 5, 18--25.

4

Virtual Screening of Acetylcholinesterase Inhibitors

Chen Dan, Pan Ya-fei, Li Chuan-jun, Xie Yun-feng and Jiang Yu-ren
Central South University,
China

1. Introduction

Alzheimer's disease (AD) is a progressive, neuro-degenerative disease, which is clinically characterized by loss of memory and progressive deficits in different cognitive domains. Widespread epidemic, long-term treatment and high medical costs have made AD a major public health problem.

AD is associated with low in vivo level of acetylcholinesterase. The consistent neuropathologic hallmark of the disorder is a massive deposit of aggregated protein degradation products, amyloid-β (Aβ) plaques and neurofibrillary tangles (Haviv et al., 2005). Even if the primary cause of AD is still speculative, Aβ aggregates are thought to be mainly responsible for the pathogenesis of the disease (Hardy & Selkoe, 2002). In recent years, significant research has been devoted to the role of free radical formation, oxidative cell damage, and inflammation in the pathogenesis of AD, providing new promising targets and validated animal models (Capsoni et al., 2000).

The major marketed drugs for the symptomatic treatment of AD are acetylcholinesterase (AChE) inhibitors, that is, tacrine (TC) (Davis & Powchik, 1995), donepezil (Bryson & Benfield, 1997), rivastigmine (Gabelli, 2003), and galantamine (Sramek et al., 2000) which inhibit AChE activity to promote an increase in the concentration and the duration of acetylcholine in the brain. However, they do not address the etiology of the disease.

The crystal structure of Torpedo California AChE (TcAChE) revealed that its active site lies at the bottom of a deep and narrow gorge (20 Å), named the "active site gorge" or "aromatic gorge" (Axelsen, 1994), the schematic can be seen in the Fig. 1. At the active site, the catalytic triad Ser200-His440-Glu327 is responsible for hydrolyzing the ester bond in ACh. At the "anionic" subsite of the active site (historically termed the "catalytic anionic site", CAS), consisting of Trp84, Tyr130, Gly199, His441 and His444 amino acid residues, adjacent to the catalytic triad, the indole side chain of the conserved residue Trp84 makes a cation-π interaction with the quaternary amino group of ACh. (Ma, 1997) A second aromatic residue, Phe330, is also involved in the recognition of ligands. The conserved residue Trp279 is the major component of a second binding site, named the peripheral "anionic" site (PAS), consisting of Tyr70 ,ASP72, Tyr121,Trp279 and Tyr334 amino acid residues, 14 Å from the active site, near the top of the gorge. (Harel, 1993) The oxyanion hole formed by the peptidic amino groups of Gly118, Gly119, Ala201 amino acid residues is another important functional unit in the esteratic subsite (Wiesner et al., 2007).

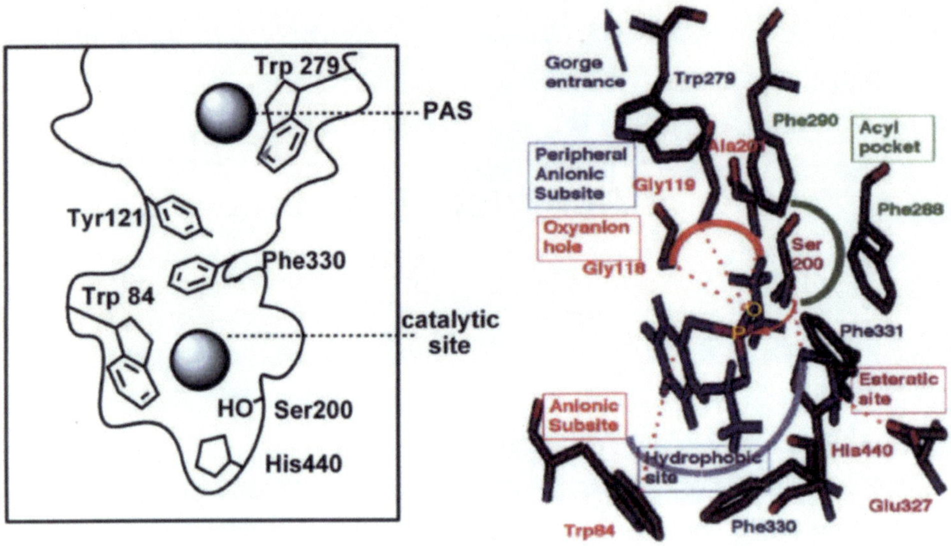

Fig. 1. The active site of AchE

Recently the peripheral anionic site (PAS) of AChE has been indicated to be involved in Aβ peptide aggregation and formed a steady compound with Aβ. On the basis of these premises, AChE inhibitors, which may alleviate cognitive deficits and behave as disease-modifying agents by inhibiting the β-amyloid (Aβ) peptide aggregation through binding to both catalytic and peripheral sites of the enzyme are becoming a new field for AD therapy.

Traditional medicine Corydalis caca has been embodied by Chinese Pharmacopoeia with the function of promoting blood circulation, relieving the pain and strengthening immunity. Ma et al. had extracted and isolated eight kinds of Tetrahydroisoquinoline alkaloids from the herb Corydalis, including Corydaline (Ma, 2008). The rigid structure containing the unit of Tetrahydroisoquinoline was shown in Fig. 2 (a). Adserson et al. found the methanol extract of Corydalis caca showing a potential inhibitory effects on the AChE activity, especially Corydaline, which is not sensible to BChE (IC50>100 μM) has the highest activity (IC50<15 μM) and selectivity among the alkaloids isolated(Adsersen et al., 2007). Because of its well-established biological properties, a type of cordalis alkaloid corydaline, which has demonstrated moderate inhibition to AChE, was used as a lead compound to obtain the action mechanism of corydaline to AChE and screen a series of its open ring derivatives by means of molecular docking and virtual screen.

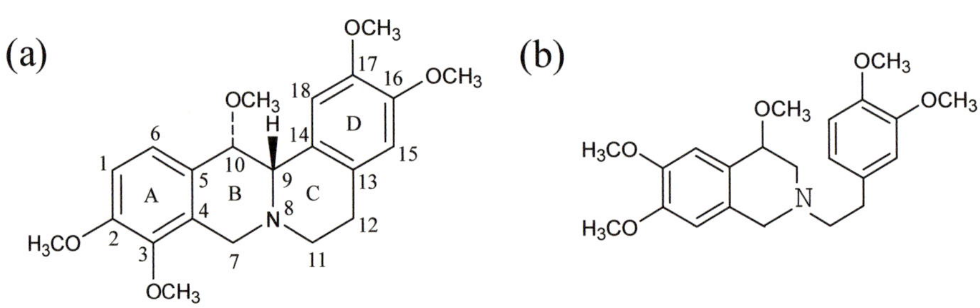

Fig. 2. Structure of Corydaline (a) and compound 7(b)

Molecular docking method (GOLD) was used by us to investigate the binding mode of corydaline with acetylcholinesterase and to screen a series of open ring derivatives with different carbon linkages and different substituent groups. Molecular Dynamics research has been done by us between the Corydaline and TcAChE with the open conformation, semi-open conformation and close conformation respectively. The best result was obtained by GOLD when corydaline was bound to the enzyme catalytic site in the open conformation. The conformation model in Fig. 5(a) indicates that phenyl ring A interacts with the phenyl group of Tyr 334 via a classic parallel π-π accumulation and that the positively charged nitrogen atom interacts with the phenyl group of Phe 330 in the hydrophobic site by the cation-π effect. Phenyl D that penetrate to the catalytic position at the bottom of the active pocket, interacts with Trp 84 via π-π effect.

Based on our former research, Yuren Jiang, et al. designed and screened a series of compounds, in which, the virtual molecule 7 was synthesized and assayed the inhibitory activity for AChE (IC50=473.3 nM • L^{-1}) (Yuren et al., 2009).The structure of virtual molecule 7 was shown in the Fig. 2 (b). Virtual screening showed that the scores of most derivatives were higher than that of corydaline, and the open ring substances with the highest scores were mainly derived from those substituted by phenoxy groups and those with 2- to 7- carbon linkages.

On account of the chemical structure of Corydaline is consisted of rigid fusedheterocycle, The length of molecule was too short to reach both the catalytic anionic site and the peripheral "anionic" site, We decided to use Corydaline as lead compound. In the reserves of Protons turn nitrogen, The C ring of Corydaline was opened in order to get derivatives that were based on the Tetrahydroisoquinoline structure. The virtual ligands with the respective substituent groups of -OH, $-OCH_3$, benzyl ect. and different length with 2- to 7- linkages were designed from alkaloids of Corydaline as potential acetylcholinesterase inhibitors. Such derivatives are able to interact with both catalytic anionic site and PAS in the TcAChE. Such design may increase the flexibility and affinity of the virtual ligands to interact with both central catalytic site and peripheral site in the TcAChE more favourably. The designed analogs of tetrahydroisoquinoline derivatives as showed in Fig. 3.

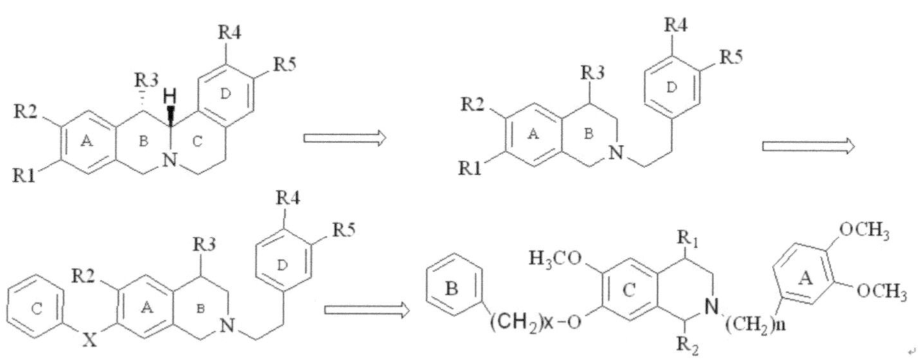

Fig. 3. The designed analogs of tetrahydroisoquinoline derivatives

2. Materials and methods

A comparison of several docking methods was carried out (Xie et al., 2006). With the purpose of investigating which docking method was more suitable for the AChE inhibitors, and the results indicated that GOLD (Jones et al., 1997) reproduced the X-ray determined conformations of known AChE inhibitors better than others. Therefore, GOLD version 3.0.1(Jones et al., 1997) was employed to probe into the binding mode between AChE and its inhibitors.

2.1 Acquisition of the AChE conformation

The crystal structure of the complex with hAChE and ligand has not been reported yet, However, Account for the sequence identity of hAChE and TcAChE is as high as 50 percent (Wiesner et al., 2007), as the Fig. 4 shows, TcAChE that obtained from the Protein Data Bank(Berman et al., 2000), can be chosen as protein acceptor. The process of the AChE conformation is to import the crystal structure of TcAChE (1EVE) to SYBYL 7.3 (Tripos Inc, 2006), delete the ligand and water molecule in the complex by using the Built/Edit module. Then add the hydrogen atom and AMBER charges to all amino acid residues by using the Biopolymer module. Save the conformation as the format of MOL2 for docking preparation.

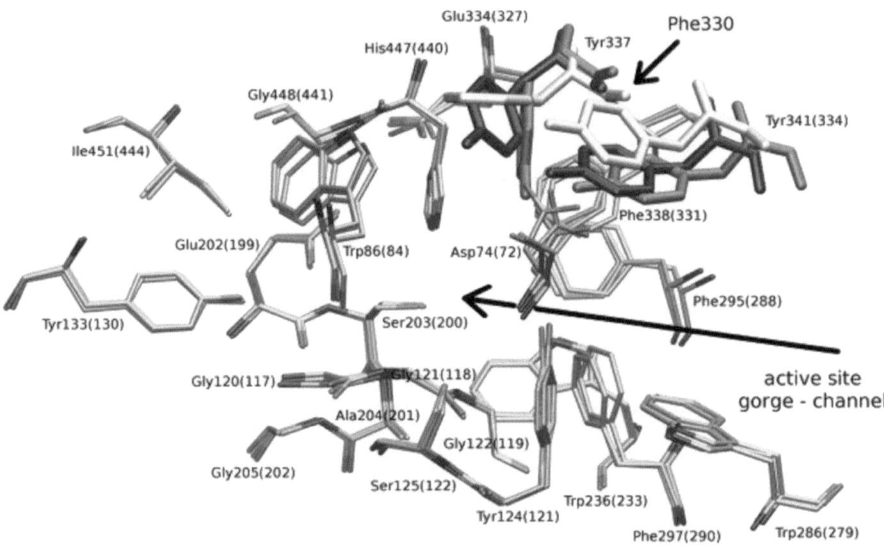

Fig. 4. 3-D alignment of human 1B41, mouse 1N5M and torpedo 1EA5 structures

2.2 Acquisition and optimization of the ligands

Corydaline and the open ring derivatives which have been designed were sketched in the Build/Edit module of SYBYL7.3.The type of the atoms and bonds in the ligands were modified to make sure they could be well- distinguished by the docking software. Then add the hydrogen atom to the ligands by using the Built/Edit module, and in the Calculation module, the charge of Gasteiger-Hukel was added to the ligands. Tripos molecular force field algorithm was chosen to modify the ligands by 3000 steps molecular mechanics optimization, Powell was chosen as iterative algorithm, and the energy gradient termination condition of the iteration was set to 0.005 kJ/(mol • nm). The key interaction truncation value was set to 1.0 nm, dielectric constant was set to 1, and other parameters were for default. Save the ligand conformations as the fomat of MOL2 for docking preparation.

2.3 Molecule docking and virtual screening

The active site was defined as all the residues within 10Å from the original ligand molecule. The default parameters of genetic algorithms (GA) were applied to search the reasonable binding conformation of these flexible ligands. The maximum number of GA runs was set to 600 for each compound. Early termination was allowed if the root mean square deviation (RMSD) of top 3 solutions are within 0.15 nm. The GOLDScore fitness function was used to evaluate the docking conformations and only energetically favourable conformations were selected for further analysis. These docked conformations were saved in MOL2 format.

2.4 Image display and data analysis

The ligand that got the highest Fitness Score in MD and the TcAChE conformation were imported into Silver at the same time, "show hydrogen bond" option was chosen to display the hydrogen bonds, "show close contracts" option was chosen to display the distance between the close atoms, and "Measure" option was chosen to calculate Hydrogen bonding Angle as well as the distance and Angle of hydrophobic interaction.

3. Results and discussion

Virtual screening showed that the scores of most derivatives were higher than that of corydaline, and the 10 open ring substances with the highest scores were mainly derived from those substituted by benzyl, methoxyl, hydroxymethyl groups, ect, and those with 2- to 7- carbon linkages. The main interactions between the ligands and the acceptor were hydrophobic interaction and hydrogen bond. The Rank and Fitness Score of the top 10 tetrahydroisoquinoline derivatives can be seen from the Table 1, in which, the Fitness score is a comprehensive evaluation of Van der Waals' force as well as hydrogen bond, considering both intramolecular and intermolecular interaction. The higher score the ligand got, represented the better affinity, the smaller IC50 and the stronger inhibitory activity. The results of molecule docking and interaction analysis showed that: all of the derivatives listed in Table 1 could interact with muti-active sites in TcAChE. In instance, the compound 8a could bind with both catalytic site and PAS at the same time, that as shown in the Fig. 5(b).

Molecular modelling obtained by GOLD suggests that, in the compound 8a, the phenyl group A of the derivatives buried within the core of the enzyme binds with the catalytic site via face-to-face π- stacking interaction (distance: 3.155Å) with Trp84. The phenyl group B reaches the peripheral site on the surface of the enzyme by face-to-face π-stacking interaction (distance: 3.225 Å) with Trp279.The protonated nitrogen atom of the tetrahydroisoquinoline moiety interacts with the phenyl group of Phe330 by cation-π interaction (distance: 4.021 Å). The phenyl group of the tetrahydroisoquinoline moiety interacts with Tyr334 by a classic parallel π-π accumulation (distance: 3.818 Å). The distance between the phenyl group A and B is 13.225 Å, which is similar to the distance that had been reported between the Trp84 and Trp279 (Harel et al., 1993).

According to the comparison of the binding mode between the Compound 8a and Corydaline, The increase has been found in both length and flexibility among the screened ligands, which guaranteed their interaction with more active sites in TcAChE, and got higher Fitness Scores and inhibitory activities.

Comp	x	n	R1	R2	Fitness score
8a	1	1	OCH_3	H	75.41
8b	1	2	OCH_3	H	74.63
8c	1	1	H	CH_2OH	72.62
8d	1	3	OCH_3	H	72.35
8e	2	1	H	CH_2OH	71.47
8f	2	1	OCH_2CH_3	CH_2OH	71.06
8g	2	1	OCH_3	CH_2OH	70.86
8h	1	2	H	CH_2OH	70.39
8i	1	2	H	H	69.40
8j	1	1	H	H	67.62
donepezil	-	-	-	-	68.53
Corydaline	-	-	-	-	56.26

Table 1. Rank and Fitness Score of the top 10 tetrahydroisoquinoline derivatives

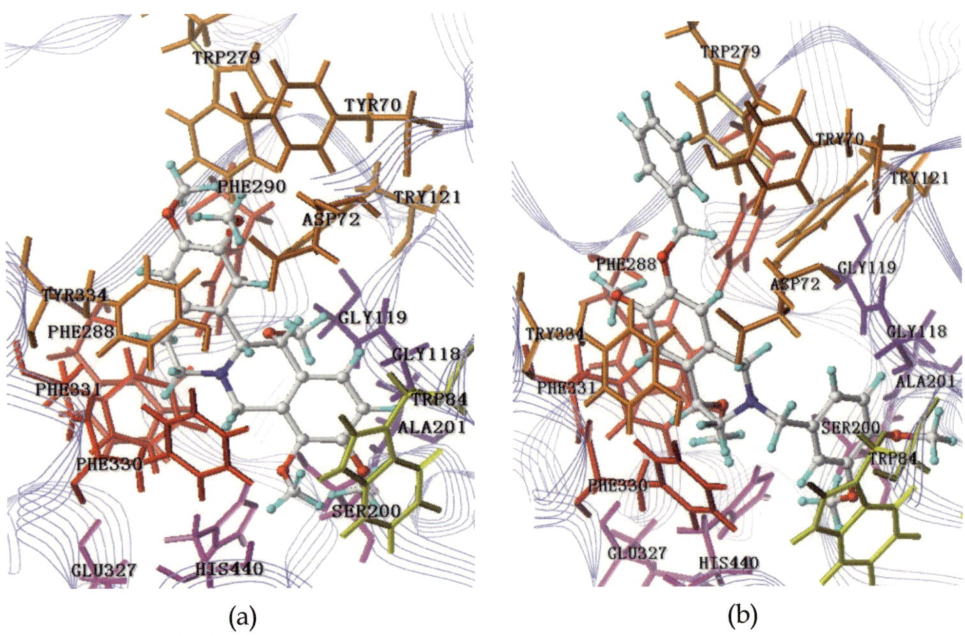

Fig. 5. Binding mode of Corydaline (a) and compound 7(b) （ball and stick） on TcAChE（stick）.The active site was marked in purple, and the peripheral "anionic" site was marked in orange.

4. Conclusion

On basis of the former research, Corydaline was used as lead compound. In the reserves of Protons turn nitrogen, the C ring of Corydaline was opened in order to get a series of derivatives. The virtual ligands with the respective substituent groups of -OH, -OCH_3, benzyl etc, and different length with 2- to 7- linkages were designed from alkaloids of Corydaline as potential acetylcholinesterase inhibitors. Such derivatives are able to interact with both active site and PAS in the TcAChE. Such design may increase the flexibility and affinity of the virtual ligands to interact with both central catalytic site and peripheral site in the TcAChE more favourably.

Molecular modelling obtained by GOLD suggests that by means of virtual screening, the compounds can bind with both catalytic anionic site and PAS in the TcAChE. The modes of binding were cation-π interaction and hydrophobic interaction. The mode was significant for the further optimization of Corydaline as well as the design of the novel following drugs.

5. Acknowledgment

The present study was supported by a grant from the National Natural Science Foundation of China (20876180).

6. References

Axelsen, P. H.; Harel, M.; Silman, I. & Sussman, J. L. (1994). Structure and dynamics of the active site gorge of acetylcholinesterase: synergistic use of molecular dynamics simulation and X-ray crystallography. *Protein Sci*, Vol. 3, No.2, pp. 188-197

Adsersen, A; Kjolbye, A.; Dall, O. & Jager, AK. (2007). Acetylcholinesterase and butyrylcholinesterase inhibitory compounds from Corydalis cava Schweigg. & Kort. *Journal of Ethnopharmacology, Vol.*113, No.1, pp. 179-182

Bryson, H. M. & Benfield, P. (1997). Donepezil. *Drugs Aging, Vol.* 10, No.3, pp. 234-239, 240-241

Berman, H. M.; Westbrook, J.; Feng, Z. & Bourne, P. (2000). The Protein Data Bank. *Nucleic acids research*, Vol. 28, No.1, pp. 235-242

Capsoni, S.; Ugolini, G.; Comparini, A. & Cattaneo, A. (2000). Alzheimer-like neurodegeneration in aged antinerve growth factor transgenic mice. *Proc. Natl. Acad. Sci.USA*, Vol. 97, No.12, pp. 6826-6831

Davis, K. L. & Powchik, P. (1995).Tacrine. *Lancet* , Vol. 345, No.8950, pp.625-630

Gabelli, C. (2003).Rivastigmine: an update on therapeutic efficacy in Alzheimer's disease and other conditions. *Curr. Med. Res.*, Vol. 19, No.2, pp.69-82

GLOD, version 3.0.1. Cambridge Crystallographic Data Centre. (2006). Cambridge, UK, 2006

Harel, M.; Schalkt, I.; Ehret-Sabatiert, L.; Bouett, F.; Goeldnert, M.; Hirtht, C.; Axelsen, P. H.; Silmanii, I. & Sussman, J. L. (1993). Quaternary ligand binding to aromatic residues in the active-site gorge of acetylcholinesterase. *Proceedings of the National Academy of Sciences of the United States of America*, Vol. 90, No.19, pp.9031-9035

Hardy, J. & Selkoe, D. J. (2002). The amyloid hypothesis of Alzheimer's disease: progress and problems on the road to therapeutics. *Science* , Vol. 297, No.5580, pp.353-356

Haviv, H.; Dawn, M. W.; Harry, M. G.;Paul, R. C.; Yuan-Ping, P.; Israel, S. & Joel, L. S. (2005). Crystal Packing Mediates Enantioselective Ligand Recognition at the

Peripheral Site of Acetylcholinesterase. *J. AM. CHEM. SOC*, Vol. 127, No.31, pp.11029-11036

Jones, G.; Willett, P.; Glen, RC.; Leach, AR. & Taylor, R. (1997). Development and validation of a genetic algorithm for flexible docking. *J Mol Biol*, Vol. 267, No.3, pp.727-748

Ma, J. C. & Dougherty, D. A. (1997). The Cationminus signpi Interaction. *Chem. ReV*, Vol. 97, No.5, pp.1303-1324

Ma, Z. Z.; Xu, W.; Jensen, N. H.; Roth, B. L.; Liu-Chen, L. Y. & Lee, D.Y.W. (2008). Isoquinoline alkaloids isolated from Corydalis yanhusuo and their binding affinities at the dopamine D1 receptor. *Molecules*, Vol. 13, No.9, pp. 2303-2312

Sramek, J. J.; Frackiewicz, E. J. & Neal, R. C. (2000). Review of the acetylcholinesterase inhibitor galanthamine. *Invest. Drugs*, Vol. 9, No.10, pp.2393-2402

Tripos Inc. (2006). Sybyl, version 7.3. St Louis, MO, USA, 2006

Wiesner, J.; Kriz, Z.; Kuca, K.; Jun, D. & Koča, J. (2007). Acetylcholinesterases-the structural similarities and differences. *Journal of Enzyme Inhibition and Medicinal Chemistry*, Vol. 22, No.4, pp.417-424

Xie, Q. ; Tang, Y.; Li, W.;Wang, X. H. & Qiu, Z. B. (2006). Investigation of the binding mode of (¨C)-meptazinol and bis-meptazinol derivative on acetylcholinesterase using a molecular docking method. *J Mol Model*, Vol. 12, pp. 390¨C

Yuren ,J.; Hui, X.; Fangjun, C. & Guanjun, M. (2009). Molecule docking and Virtual screening for Acetylcholinesterases inhibitor Corydaline. *Acta Physico Chimica Sinica*, Vol. 52, No.7, pp. 1379-1384

5

Computational Virtual Screening Towards Designing Novel Anticancer Drugs

Po-Yuan Chen[1,2]
[1]*Department of Biological Science and Technology, China Medical University, Taichung, Taiwan,*
[2]*Brain Research Centre, University of British Columbia, Vancouver,*
[1]*Republic of China*
[2]*Canada*

1. Introduction

Generally speaking, Docking is most popular and critical issue in this research field, because it contains most important information both Ligands (Drugs) and Receptors (it can be intracellular protein, trans-membrane protein or extracellular protein). However, when the ligand's information is not sufficient, it needs other calculation strategies to design and "modify" the ligands, and theoretically improve the drug effects, and that is called *De Novo* Evolution Drug Design. Current methods for structure-based drug design can be divided roughly into two categories. The first category is about "finding" ligands for a given receptor, which is usually referred as database searching. In this case, a large number of potential ligand molecules are screened to find those fitting the binding pocket of the receptor. This method is usually referred as structure-based drug design. The key advantage of database searching is that it saves synthetic effort to obtain new lead compounds. Another category of structure-based drug design methods is about "building" ligands, which is usually referred as receptor-based drug design. In this case, ligand molecules are built up within the constraints of the binding pocket by assembling small pieces in a stepwise manner. These pieces can be either individual atoms or molecular fragments. The key advantage of such a method is that novel structures, not contained in any database, can be suggested. These techniques are raising much excitement to the drug design community. Above two computational methods, the first is called virtual screening by Docking (the drugs are well prepared and need to be screen out the most suitable candidates), and the other is *De.Novo* Evolution Drug Design (*De Novo* means "creates" or "building" ligands) [1-3]. However, when the targeting protein is unclear, or the factors are complicated, QSAR method is implemented to help user solving these problems. Because QSAR method just needs ligands structures and IC_{50} datasets to unveil an unknown novel drugs. Finally, when both of Ligands and Receptors are unknown, Homology Modeling is the only method for dealing with this problem. By using Homology Modeling, the Receptors 1-D sequences similarities can be used as a tool to reconstruct the 3-D structures.

2. Methods and materials

Docking small molecules (ligands) into larger protein molecules (receptors) is a complex and difficult task. Docking programs include CDOCKER, LibDock, and **LigandFit**. Here, I introduce **LigandFit** for this research because it bases on an initial shape matched to the binding site and it is easier to observe the interaction of the ligand and the protein.

There are two major parts of the **LigandFit** docking:

1. Specify the region of the receptor to use as the binding site for docking. Site partitioning may be applied to select parts of the binding site during docking.
2. Dock ligands to the specified site. This part consists of the following steps:
   a. Conformational search to generate candidate ligand conformations for docking;
   b. Compare the ligand shape and protein binding site shape by computing their size of possession;
   c. Minimize the rigid body energy of the candidate ligand pose/conformation by using the Dockscore calculation.

In the following steps, we discard the water (because it will be complicated to the calculations) and ligand from the receptor protein, and calculate the score for the ligand docking to protein. Check the interacting force between the receptor protein and drugs (Fig. 1).

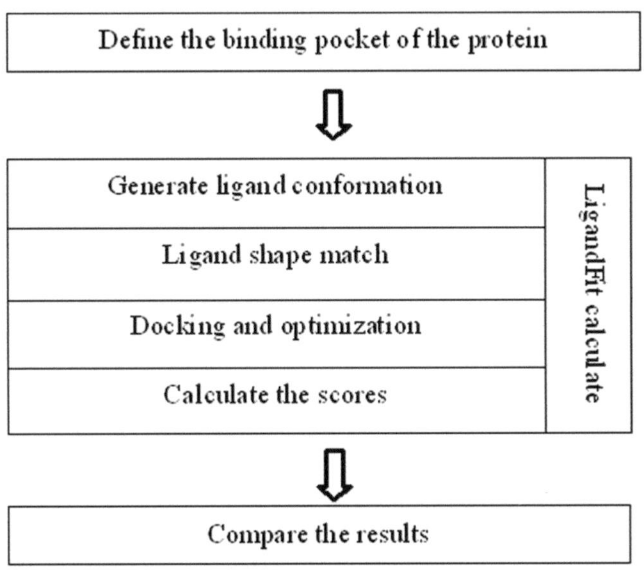

Fig. 1. The procedure of **LigandFit** Docking procedure

LigandFit: Docking and Score using Accelrys Software

The score functions in the Discovery Studio 2.5 which we used were Dock Score, PLP1, PLP2 and PMF. Candidate ligand poses are evaluated and prioritized according to the Dock Score function. There are two types of Dock Score. One is based on a force-field approximation, the other on the Piecewise Linear Potential function (PLP).

$$\text{DockScore (forcefield)} = -\,(\text{ligand/receptor interaction energy} + \text{ligand internal energy}) \quad (1)$$

$$\text{DockScore(PLP)} = - \text{(PLP potential)} \quad (2)$$

As shown in *Equation1*, there are two energy terms in the force-field version of Dock Score, internal energy of the ligand and the interaction energy of the ligand with the receptor. The interaction energy is taken as the sum of the van der Waals energy and electrostatic energy. The computation of the interaction energy can be quite time consuming. To reduce the time needed for this calculation, a grid-based estimation of the ligand/receptor interaction energy is employed [4].

The van der Waals component of the force-field interaction energy typically exhibits a steep rise at short interatomic distances, which can have undesirable consequences in the context of ligand-receptor docking. In particular, the combination of approximating the receptor structure as rigid and limited sampling of ligand conformational space tends to overly penalize poses with "mild" short contacts between the ligand and receptor, due to the "hard" nature of the van der Waals potential as defined in most standard force-fields.

To overcome this tendency, a softened form of the van der Waals potential is employed with the Dock Score function. This softened potential rises to a large but finite value at zero interatomic separation. To maintain a proper balance between electrostatics and van der Waals, the electrostatic energy is also softened to prevent it from dominating the van der Waals energy at short separations.

The internal energy of the ligand is computed when using the force-field version of Dock Score. The purpose of including the internal energy is to avoid ligand conformations with bad internal non-bond clashes. By default, only the standard (not softened) van der Waals energy is used for the ligand internal energy. Including electrostatic energy as part of the ligand internal energy is optionally available.

The PLP version of Dock Score uses the PLP1 function, because the functional form of PLP1 allows it to be readily represented with a grid-based approach. The PLP2 function has an angular dependence on hydrogen bonding interactions making its representation with a grid considerably more difficult.

In the PLP1 score function, there are four atom types as following: **(1)** hydrogen bond donor only, **(2)** hydrogen bond acceptor only, **(3)** both hydrogen bond donor and acceptor, and **(4)** non-polar. When PLP1 is the docking scores function, the internal energy is calculated for each ligand conformation that the ligand is in the binding site [5].

In the PLP2 score function [6], the atom typing remains the same as in the PLP1 score function. In addition, an atomic radius is assigned to each atom expect for hydrogen [7].

The PMF score function was developed based on statistical analysis of the 3D structures of the protein-ligand complex [8]. They were found to correlate well with protein-ligand binding free energy while being fast and simple to calculate. The scores are calculated by summing pairwise interaction terms over all interatomic pairs of the receptor-ligand complex. The score function of Dock Score is the default function in the Discovery Studio 2.5.

All the simulations were also applied by CHARMM (Chemistry at Harvard Macromolecular Mechanics) Force-field. CHARMM was parameterized by experimental data. It has been used widely for simulations ranging from small molecules to solvated complexes of large biological macromolecules. CHARMM performs well over a broad range of calculations and simulations, including minima, time-dependent dynamic behavior, and barriers to rotation, vibrational frequencies, and free energy. CHARMM uses a flexible and comprehensive energy function:

$$E_{(pot)} = E_{bond} + E_{torsion} + E_{oop} + E_{elect.} + E_{vdW} + E_{constraint} + E_{user}$$

Where, the out-of-plane (OOP) angle is an important torsion. The van der Waals term is derived from rare-gas potentials, and the electrostatic term can be scaled to mimic solvent effects. Hydrogen-bond energy is not included as a separate term as in AMBER. Instead, hydrogen-bond energy is implicit in the combination of van der Waals and electrostatic terms [9].

3. Research highlight

In this section, I summarize some of my research works published in Journal of Life Sciences and IEEE *International Conference on Bioinformatics and Bioengineering*, which includes anti-lung cancer and anti-oral cancer research, as illustrated as follows:

3.1 Anti-lung cancer research

The purpose of this research is to use computer docking and screening for the new type MEK1 inhibitor in lung cancer cells through the initiation of receptor tyrosine kinase and Mitogen-activated protein kinase pathway. The influence of lung cancer cell propagation suppressing by the combination of MEK protein and ATP was also discussed. A more active and potential drug molecule which can effectively lower the cost of developing lung cancer drugs can be proposed through the use of bioinformatics software and a series of data comparison, screening, and statistical analysis[10, 11].

In this paper, "Computational Screening of Novel Mitogen-activated Protein Kinase Kinase-1 (MEK1) Inhibitors by Docking and Scoring" [11], we discuss the MEK1 inhibitors by using **LigandFit** method to evaluate the affinity of the drug candidates (**LIGANDS**) towards the target **Protein** (Receptors, MEK1). The best docking poses analysis can be illustrated by Fig. 2 [11]. In this figure, we can reveal which interaction forces are the critical roles in **LIGANDS** and **Protein.**

There are several factors affecting the practical activity, such as the amino acids: LYS97, ASP190 in MEK protein, which are located at the entrance of the **PROTEINs**. When the **LIGAND** enter into the **PROTEIN**, some atoms of the **LIGAND** will bond to the entrance amino acids, moreover PHE209 which is at the terminal of the cavity will produce π-stacking force or H-BOND bonding, and the **LIGANDs** will not leave the **PROTEINs**. The **LIGANDs** of the high activity group almost have these characters, which will effectively inhibit the MEK PROTEIN. When talking about the **LIGANDs** of the low activity group, they enter a small way into the **PROTEIN**, and can easily leave the **PROTEIN**. PHE209 at the terminal of the cavity of the **PROTEIN** will affect the activity. The authors found the **LIGAND** of the high activity group had the aromatic group at the end of the molecule. So they would arise from the π-stacking force. The medium activity **LIGANDs** formed a small-stacking force. For the low activity **LIGANDs**, they would not form stacking force because they have no aromatic groups [11].

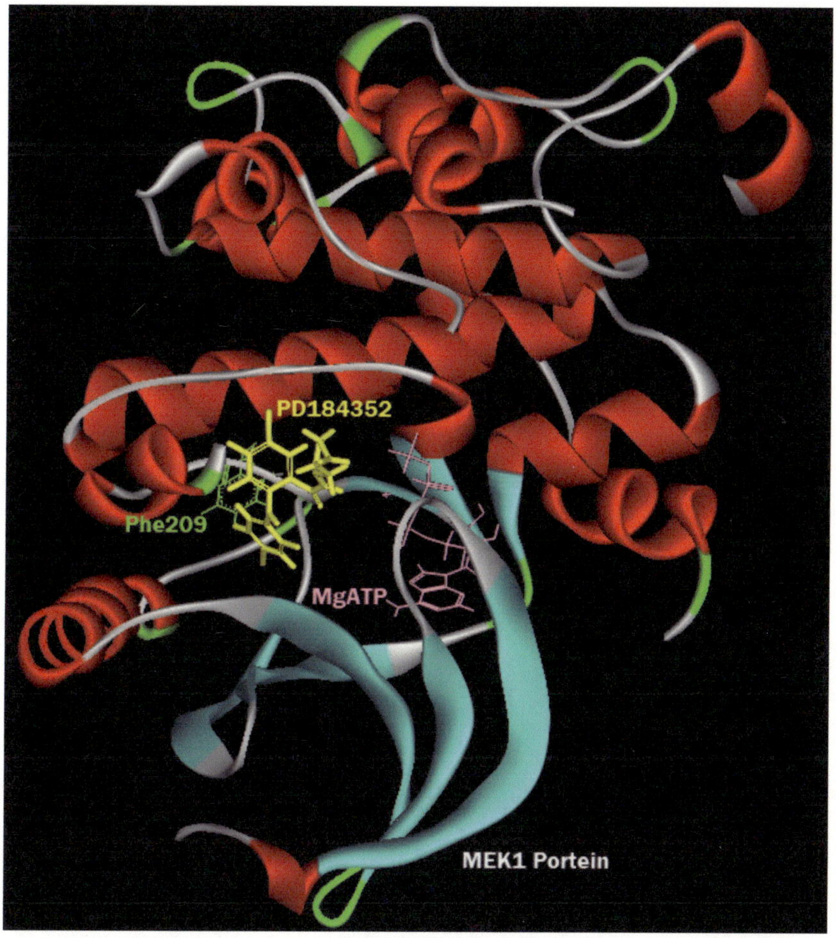

Fig. 2.A PD184352 interacts with the PROTEIN and produces non-competitively with MgATP. It migrates into the PROTEIN and produces HBOND with MgATP and arouses a π stacking force with PHE209. PD184352 holds tightly with the PROTEIN and the MEK1 PROTEIN will lose its function. [11]

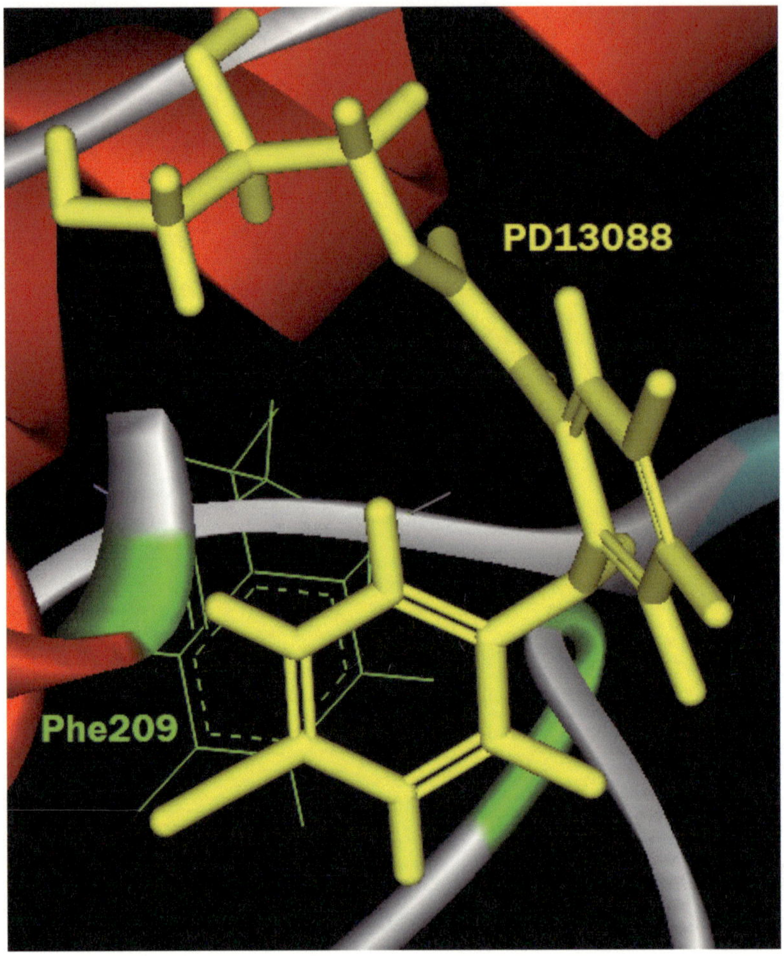

Fig. 2.B This figure shows the location of the aromatic group of PHE209 and the aromatic group of PD13088. It reveals they probably have a π stacking force. [11]

3.2 Anti-oral cancer research

This research paper "Predication the suppressing human oral cancer cell line by curcumin through the research of Fas receptor" [12] which is expected to calculate the activity of *Curcumin* to Fas receptor. Fas receptor is a key receptor which commonly mechanisms caused to oral cancer. The pharmaceutical activity are evaluate by the score from docking procedure perform by simulation program.

The occurrence rate and death rate of oral cancer increased year by year according to the statistic value from Department of Health. The statistical report published by DOH in 2009 indicates that the death rate of oral cancer rank number 6 in Taiwan among all 10 kinds of cancer and the occurrence rate rank number 4 in male among 10 kinds of cancer. These values persist very high in recent years. Tongue cancer and buccal cancer are the cancer with highest frequency in oral cancer. These two cancers take almost 90% of oral cancer and tongue cancer take 60% among all which is the highest. The effect of treating tongue cancer is far less than buccal cancer which makes the five year survival rate of oral cancer decrease gradually. Curcumin is able to activate the apoptosis pathway to make cancer cell apoptosis and achieve the anti-cancer effect. The purpose of this research is to simulate the pharmaceutical activity and evaluate the degree of activity to determine: (1) whether curcumin is able to activate cell apoptosis to oral cancer cells? (2) Is the pharmaceutical activity of curcumin to oral cancer cells higher than those medicines on market?

Fas receptor (FasR) is a kind of death receptor on cell surface which can initiate the programmed cell death (cell apoptosis) through extrinsic pathway. Another one is the intrinsic pathway (mtirochondira). These are two types of cell apoptosis. FasR can also be called as CD95 which is the member of superfamilty of Apo-1 and TNF receptor [13, 14]. FasR is located on the 10th chromosome in human and 19th chromosome in rate. There are similar sequences in most mammal chromosomes [15]. The death-inducing signaling complex (DISC) formed by Fas can combine with receptor (FasL). FasL trimer makes the adjacent FasR to shape into trimer on the membrane and active the DISC below to attract and combine with Fas associsted death dimain(FADD). FADD will further attarct pro-caspase 8 for combination and cut the pro-caspase 8 into caspase 8. The caspase 8 will further cut and activate pro-caspase, therefore the caspase cascase magnifying effect is aroused to reinforce the activation of caspase 3. The caspase 3 will destruct the structural proteins such as cytokeletal protein and finish the apoptosis (reference: Eksp Klin Farmakol. 2010 Dec;73(12):44-9).

Curcumin, which is a kind of yellowish pigment extract from roots of turmeric. 70% of Curcumin is composed of curcuminoid which takes 3%~6% of turmeric (http://curcumin-turmeric.net/). The application of curcumin is far from now which curcumin were used as nature pigment in food industry. Beside, curcumin is stable to reductant and with good coloring ability but sensitive to light, heat and iron ions. The major application the coloring for canned food, sausages, and stewed soy sauce produce. Curcumin is also applied as acid-base indicator [pH 7.8 (yellow)- 9.2 (reddish brown)] (http://www.lookchem.cn/4150/productproperty.html). Curcumin have critical value and pharmaceutical action such as decreasing the blood fat, anti-oxidation, anti-inflammatory, and anti-atherosclerosis. Research in 2004 even found that curcumin can be use to suppress the activity of HIV-1 integrase and applied in AIDS clinical trial [16]. Beside the above functions, curcumin is also proved to have the pharmaceutical activity to anticancer and the effect of suppressing carcinoma have been verified repeatedly during many animal experiments [17, 18].

This research is to calculate and simulate the pharmaceutical activity of anticancer effects of *Curcumin* to oral cancer and get quality evaluation results. The preliminary results are listed as figures and tables below. The receptor applied is curcumin-derivatives: bisdemethoxy curcumin; target protein: FAS/FADD death domain assembly (*Protein PDB ID*: 3OQ9) to perform Docking and Scoring:

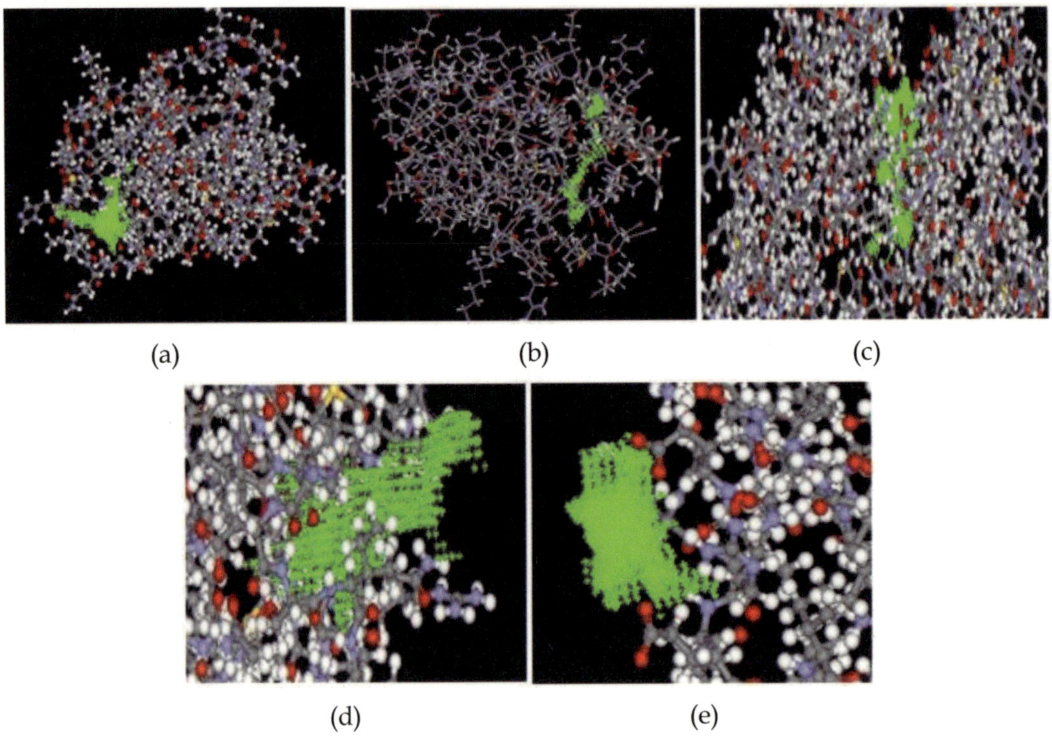

Fig. 3. (a) Bind Site-A & Ligand poses (I) (b) Bind Site-A & Ligand poses (III) (c) Bind Site-B & Ligand poses (I) (d) Bind Site-B & Ligand poses (II) (e) Bind Site-B & Ligand poses (III)

Bind Site-A & Ligand poses (I)			Bind Site-A & Ligand poses (III)			Bind Site-B & Ligand poses (I)		
Name	Index	DOCK_SCORE	Name	Index	DOCK_SCORE	Name	Index	DOCK_SCORE
Molecule-1	1	36.04	Molecule-1	1	24.895	Molecule-1	1	18.071
Molecule-1	2	32.879	Molecule-1	2	17.943	Molecule-1	2	17.132
Bind Site-B & Ligand poses (II)			Bind Site-B & Ligand poses (III)					
Name	Index	DOCK_SCORE	Name	Index	DOCK_SCORE			
Molecule-1	1	24.895	Molecule-1	1	39.984			
Molecule-1	2	17.943	Molecule-1	2	39.777			

Table 1. Docking Score data

4. Conclusions

In this chapter, I introduce the simple docking method: **LigandFit.** Without consider the water-containing environment (water free), and flexible situations (**PROTEINs** vibration), the estimations will be worthy of discussion. However, because of its fast screening and effective for most Receptor cases, it can be applied to many anti-cancer drugs candidate virtual screening at many situations.

5. Acknowledgement

This work was supported by a grant from China Medical University (CMU95-173, CMU96-107). The corresponding authors would like to thank their parents, all colleagues and friends who contributed to this study. We thank the editor and series editor for constructive criticisms and comments.

6. References

[1] Wang, R., Gao, Y., Lai, L. (2000), "LigBuilder: A Multi-Purpose Program for Structure-Based Drug Design". *Journal of Molecular Modeling* 6 (7-8): 498–516.

[2] Schneider, G., Fechner, U. (2005), "Computer-based de novo design of drug-like molecules". *Nat Rev Drug Discov* 4 (8): 649–663.

[3] Jorgensen, W. L. (2004), "The many roles of computation in drug discovery". *Science* 303 (5665): 1813–1818.

[4] Venkatachalam, C. M., Jiang, X., Oldfield, T. Waldman, M. (2003), "LigandFit: a novel method for the shape-directed rapid docking of ligands to protein active sites". *Journal of Molecular Graphics and Modelling*. 21(4), 289-307.

[5] Gehlhaar, D. K., Verkhivker, G. M., Rejto, P. A., Sherman, C. J., Fogel, D. B., Fogel, L. J., Freer, S. T. (1995), "Molecular Recognition of the Inhibitor AG-1343 by HIV-1 Protease: Conformationally Flexible Docking by Evolutionary Programming". *Chemistry & Biology* 2, 317.

[6] Gehlhaar, D. K., Bouzida, D., Rejto, P. A. (1999). *Rational Drug Design: Novel Methodology and Practical Applications* ; Parrill, L.; Rami Reddy, M; Series title: ACS symposium series, 719; American Chemical Society: Washington, DC., 292-311.

[7] Bouzida, D., Arthurs S., *et al*, (1999). Thermodynamics and kinetics of ligand-protein binding studied with the weighted histogram analysis method and simulated annealing, *Pac Symp Biocomput*, , 426-437.

[8] Muegge, I. and Martin, Y. C. (1999), "A general and fast scoring function for protein-ligand interactions: a simplified potential approach", *J Med Chem*, 42, 791-804.

[9] Brooks, B.R., Bruccoleri, R.E., Olafson, B.D., States, D.J., Swaminathan, S., Karplus, M. (1983), "CHARMM: A program for macromolecular energy, minimization, and dynamics calculations". *J Comp Chem* 4 (2): 187–217.

[10] Chen, P. Y., Jhuo, M. D., Hsu, W. T., Shih, T. C., Cheng T. H., (2009), "The MAPK Signal Pathway Research and New Drug Discovery", *2009 Ninth IEEE International Conference on Bioinformatics and Bioengineering*, 370-373.

[11] Chen, P. Y., Hong, H. J., Jhuo, M. D., Cheng, T. H., Hsu, W. T., Wu, C. H., Ou, C. Y., Yui, Y. T., Lin, J. P., Chung, J. G., (2011), "Computational Screening of Novel Mitogen-activated Protein Kinase Kinase-1(MEK1) Inhibitors by Docking and Scoring", *Journal of Life Sciences*, 5, 434-442.

[12] Chen, P. Y., Wu, Y. C., Cheng, T. H., Shih, T. C., Tsai, C. T., Wu, C. H., Hua, T. Y. Huang, Y. Y., Cheng, C. H., Fan, M. J. (2011), "Predication the suppressing human oral cancer cell line by curcumin through the research of Fas receptor", *2011 Ninth IEEE International Conference on Bioinformatics and Bioengineering, accepted.*

[13] Neumann, L., Pforr, C., Beaudouin, J., Pappa, A., Fricker, N., Krammer, P.H., Lavrik, I.N., Eils, R. (2010). "Dynamics within the CD95 death-inducing signaling complex decide life and death of cells", *Molecular Systems Biology*. 6, 352.
[14] Nagata, S. (1997), "Apoptosis by death factor", *Cell*. 88, 355-65.
[15] Cascino, I., Papoff, G., Eramo, A., Ruberti, G. (1996), "Soluble Fas/Apo-1 splicing variants and apoptosis", *Frontiers in Bioscience*. 1, d12-8.
[16] Padma TV. Turmeric can combat malaria, cancer virus and HIV. SciDev.net. 2005-03-11
[17] Aggarwal, B. B., Shshodia, S. (2006), "Molecular targets of dietary agents for prevention and therapy of cancer", *Biochemical Pharmacology- Elsevier*. 71, 1397–421.
[18] Choi, H., Chun, Y.S., Kim, S.W., Kim, M.S., Park, J. W.. (2006), "Curcumin Inhibits Hypoxia-Inducible Factor-1 by Degrading Aryl Hydrocarbon Receptor Nuclear Translocator: A Mechanism of Tumor Growth Inhibition. Molecular Pharmacology", *American Society for Pharmacology and Experimental Therapeutics*. 70, 1664–71.